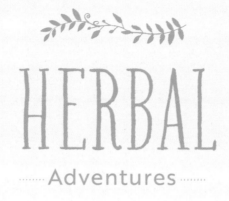

HERBAL

·····Adventures·····

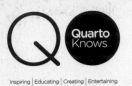
First published in 2018 by Young Voyageur Press, an imprint of The Quarto Group, 401 Second Avenue North, Suite 310, Minneapolis, MN 55401 USA.
T (612) 344-8100 F (612) 344-8692 www.QuartoKnows.com

Young Voyageur Press titles are also available at discount for retail, wholesale, promotional, and bulk purchase. For details, contact the Special Sales Manager by email at specialsales@quarto.com or by mail at The Quarto Group, Attn: Special Sales Manager, 401 Second Avenue North, Suite 310, Minneapolis, MN 55401 USA.

10 9 8 7 6 5 4 3 2 1

ISBN: 978-0-7603-6051-4

Library of Congress Cataloging-in-Publication Data
Names: Jepson Wolf, Rachel, 1973- author.
Title: Herbal adventures : backyard excursions and kitchen creations for kids and their families / Rachel Jepson Wolf.
Description: Minneapolis, MN : Young Voyageur Press, an imprint of The Quarto Group, 2018. | Includes bibliographical references and index.
Identifiers: LCCN 2018012188 | ISBN 9780760360514 (hc : alk. paper)
Subjects: LCSH: Materia medica, Vegetable. | Medicinal plants. | Herbs--Therapeutic use.
Classification: LCC RS164 .J47 2018 | DDC 615.3/21--dc23
LC record available at https://lccn.loc.gov/2018012188

DISCLAIMER

Acquiring Editor: Thom O'Hearn
Project Manager: Alyssa Lochner
Art Director: Laura Drew
Page Design: Sussner Design
Layout: Diana Boger

Printed in China

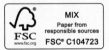

MIX
Paper from responsible sources
FSC® C104723

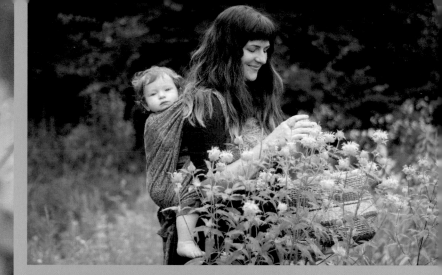

HERBAL

·····Adventures·····

Backyard Excursions
and Kitchen Creations
for Kids and
Their Families

RACHEL JEPSON WOLF

Foreword by Amanda Blake Soule

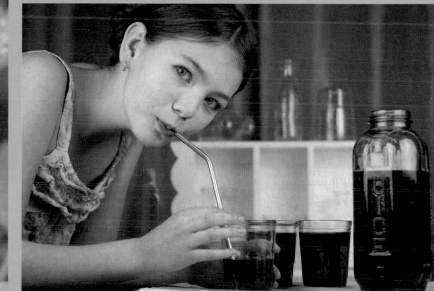

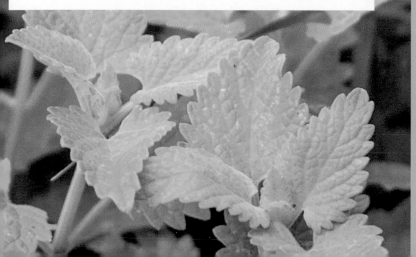

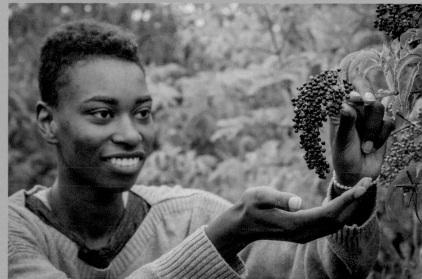

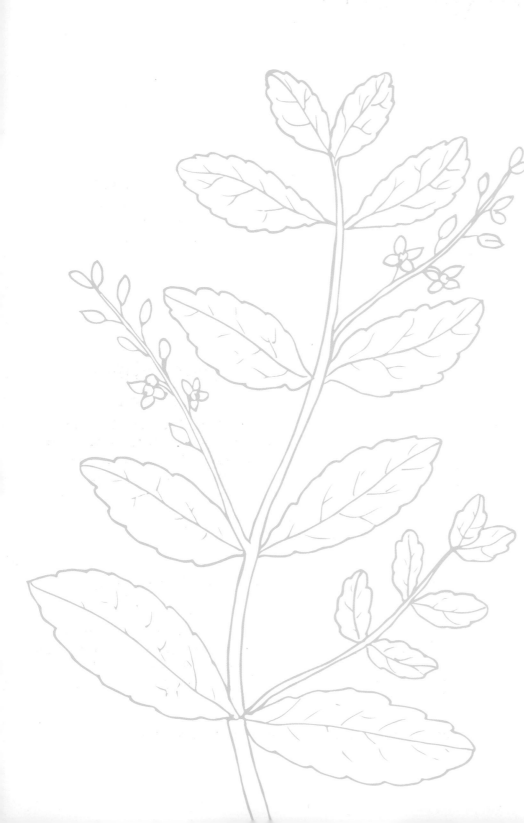

CONTENTS

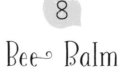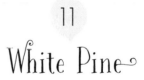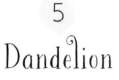

FOREWORD

A Note to Parents from Amanda Blake Soule

So many precious childhood memories take place in nature—whether deep in a forest or in an urban city park. Growing up, my own neighborhood was suburban, but it had a little patch of wild. A potential house lot, never developed, became a place where the neighborhood children would run and play. We had an elaborate fort system in those brambles where we passed long summer days with one another. We all learned (by necessity) to identify and stay away from the poison ivy. Over time, we built our knowledge; we discovered things such as where and when the milkweed could be found—and that the butterflies would visit it. I now know that plot was just one acre, but it felt enormous, and oh so important, as a child.

Today, my own children have a forty-acre plot in which they explore, scattered with forts and treehouses amidst the brambles and the poison ivy (which they can all identify). It has become one of the places where our family connects. Though we spend a good deal of time working in the woods—clearing trail and cutting down firewood—there's more that happens on each and every walk. In these woods, we find many of the earth's precious plants, gently harvest them, and bring them back inside with us for health, wellness, medicinal, and nutritional use. Each year, we learn a little bit more about what plants thrive in our neck of the woods and what they can offer us.

Just as important, foraging is an activity during which our family spends time together free from the distractions of busy modern lives. Our focus turns to our surroundings. We must pay careful attention, slowing down to notice each seasonal change, and in the end we find not just plants . . . but peace.

Beyond locating your own patch of wilderness, where do you start? It can be daunting to find what you're looking for, and tough to know what to do with the herbs once you have them in hand. Fortunately, in these pages, Rachel provides everything you'll need for a lovely family walk "into the woods." You'll find photos and information to help you confidently identify plants, as well as easy-to-craft projects. The recipes are accessible and useful to all members of the family.

By following her lead, we are empowered to heal our bodies and connect with the earth and one another. What a lifelong gift we can give our children in these simple acts.

Cheers to the herbal adventures ahead!

—Amanda Blake Soule
author of *The Creative Family*
and editor of *Taproot* magazine

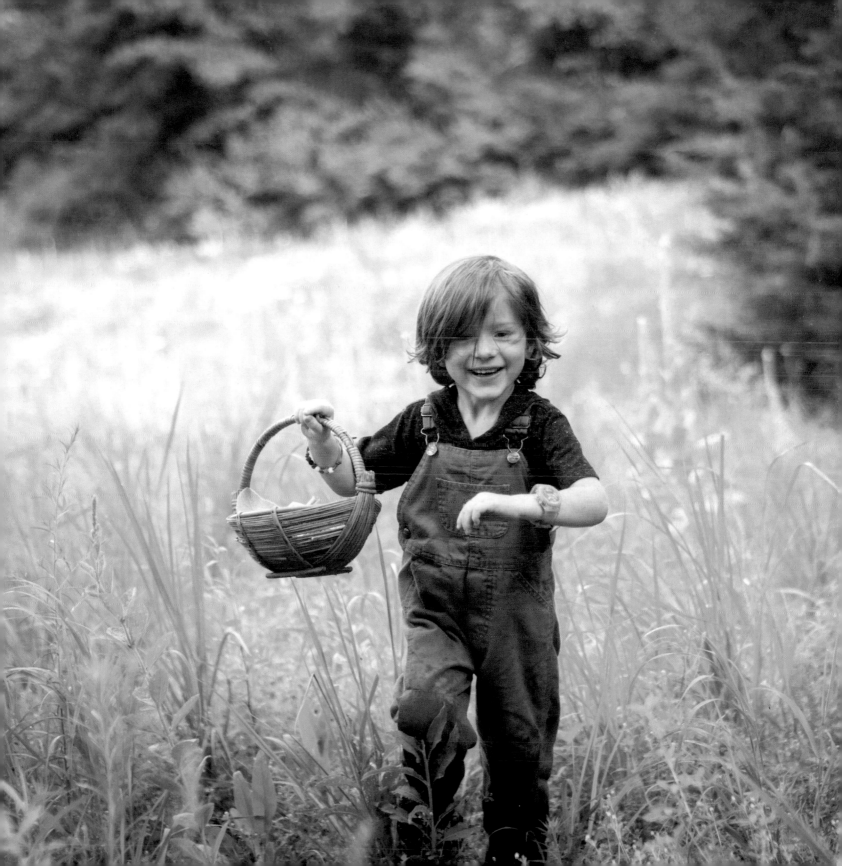

INTRODUCTION

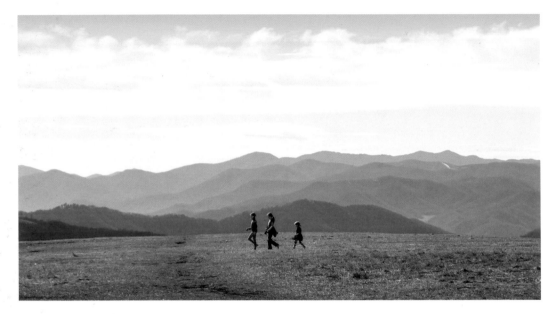

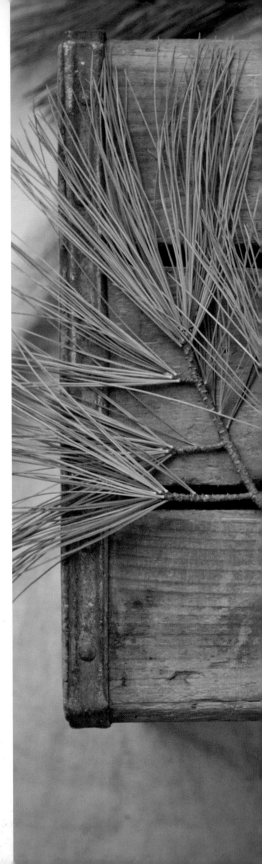

When our great-great-grandmothers were tending to their families' needs, they looked no further than their own backyards for remedies to bring comfort and healing. Here they found the herbs they needed to treat a cough, soothe a sore throat, calm a diaper rash, or quiet a fussy baby.

They knew which plants were appropriate for which conditions, and this knowledge was fine-tuned to suit their region and to their families' needs. Like favorite family recipes, this wisdom was passed down generation after generation. Each kitchen herbalist who inherited it made refinements and additions based on their own experiences, intuition, and preferences.

But somewhere along the way, as we moved into a more industrialized culture, this knowledge was misplaced. Backyard weeds-as-medicine fell out of favor and were replaced by over-the-counter syrups, pills, and creams.

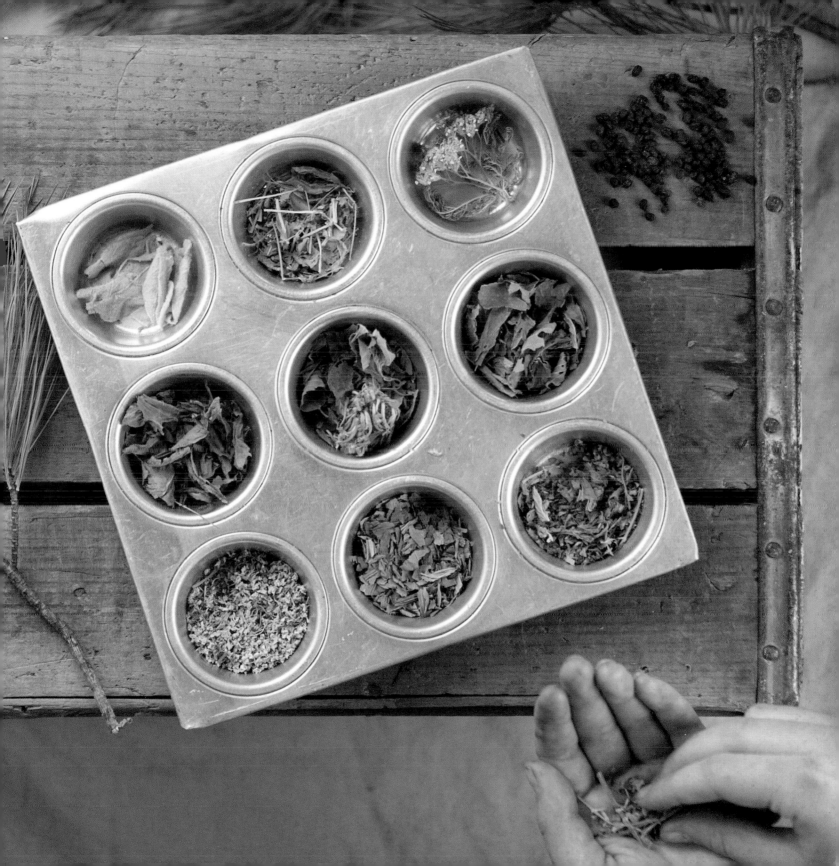

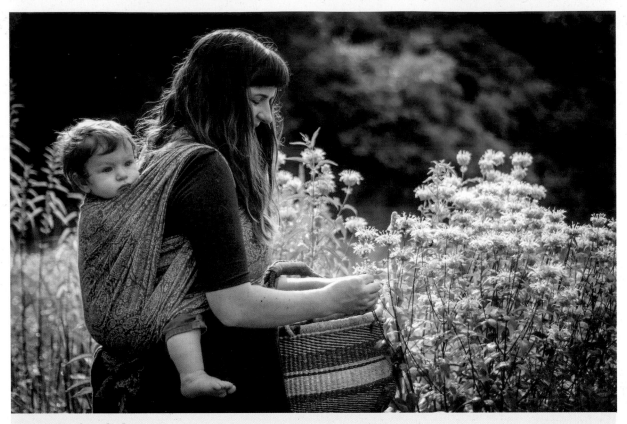

Foraging bee balm

Eventually, as a culture, we forgot that homemade remedies are effective, affordable, and easy to make. We forgot how well they work with our bodies, triggering our immune and nervous systems to heal themselves. We forgot how it feels to deeply nourish and heal the body, often from the inside out.

But today we're beginning to remember.

One child and one adult at a time, we're picking up what was forgotten. We're learning the old ways once more and reclaiming our green legacy. We are turning back to the plants again and asking them to share their secrets.

Had we grown up in a different time, our childhood days may have been spent in the garden and the forest alongside a parent or grandparent, helping forage herbs for both food and remedies. We would know the plants like we know old friends and readily harvest one for a cough, another for a cut, and another for sore muscles. Yet today, many of us are unsure where to begin.

By writing this book, I hope that everyone—parents and children alike—will have a chance to regain a bit of that misplaced wisdom. Wisdom that was yours all along. These plants and these pages mark the starting point of an herbal adventure that will take you as far as you wish to go!

Wild chamomile

What is an herbal remedy?

Throughout this book we'll explore "herbal remedies" and "herbal medicines." But what exactly do those terms mean? An herbal remedy or medicine is simply a treatment for an injury or illness made from the leaves, berries, roots, flowers, or bark of a plant. These remedies come in many different forms, from teas and syrups to oils and salves.

For any adult who has felt a bit lost in learning the names (much less the uses!) of common wild plants, for any child who has lain on the cool earth watching for fairies and listening to the wind, for any of us who has felt the calm comfort that nature can bring, may this book be a key that opens doors of knowledge and wonder and brings you the satisfaction of self-sufficiency.

As you get to know the ten plants featured in this book and learn how to use them to make syrups, teas, treats, and more, your eyes will open to the vast world of herbs and remedies just beyond your back door. You're setting off with this book in hand, but this is only the first step of your journey! This discovery will take you far beyond these pages as you set off on a path of learning, experimentation, and curious exploration of your own making.

In the backyard, the garden, and the kitchen, you'll happily reclaim this forgotten knowledge as you learn and create side by side with your loved ones. And although today you might not know which plant to pick from the yard for a bee sting, or which to brew for the common cold, you soon will.

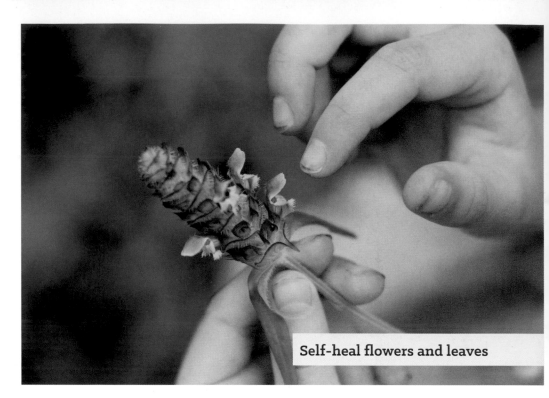

Self-heal flowers and leaves

My hope is that this knowledge becomes second nature to you, something that you carry with you wherever you go and readily share with your family and friends. Nothing would be more delightful than to know that this knowledge becomes a part of you forever.

Before We Begin

Notes for Parents and Caregivers

Exploring herbs for the first time is an adventure at any age! And although I've written the chapters that follow with children in mind, this book is the perfect introduction to herbs for parents and other grownups as well.

Because it is a book for beginners, I have attempted to keep things simple on the pages that follow. Rather than overwhelm you with dozens of uses for each herb, I've focused in on just two or three uses for each plant. However, that focus is certainly not the plant's only gift! Further research will reveal a plethora of uses for the herbs found in this book, as well as for plants you discover beyond these pages. (The resources section is rich with recommendations of other books to add to your library that will allow you to dig even deeper into the world of herbal remedies.) Here are the important things to keep in mind as you read this book:

Better together:

Most of the recipes and crafts I have shared are designed for ages six and up, with some adult help here and there. Since paints, scissors, knives, stoves, and many other mishaps-waiting-to-happen are involved in most of these projects, your close supervision of younger children is strongly encouraged—and implicit in the instructions! While many of the recipes can easily be undertaken by older kids with minimal guidance, why not play along as well? You may discover a new side of plants—or yourself—that you never expected.

Contraindications:

If you or someone you are giving remedies to has any medical conditions or is taking any medications, always check carefully for any contraindicated herbs, and talk to your health-care provider before embarking on a new herbal protocol. Many herbal formulas are not recommended for pregnant women simply because of the lack of information on how the herbs might affect mother or child, so use extra caution if pregnant or nursing. And due to the presence of botulism spores in honey (both raw and pasteurized), honey is not recommended in any amount to children under one year of age. While these spores are harmless to older children and adults, they are dangerous for babies in their first year. Common contraindications are noted for the recipes in this book; however, I encourage you to consult your health-care provider if you have any medical conditions or are currently taking any medications.

Go slow:

Any time you introduce a new herb or formula, begin slowly. Listen to how your body reacts when you take or apply it, and never continue using an herb that you have a negative reaction to.

Spot test:

For those with sensitive skin, spot-testing topical remedies can be helpful. To spot-test, simply apply a small amount of any new remedy to the inside forearm at bedtime, and cover with a bandage. The next day, remove the bandage and examine the skin. If the spot where the remedy was applied is red or irritated, the remedy is not an appropriate choice and use should be discontinued.

Plant play:

In addition to exploring specific plants and remedies, this book is peppered with a variety of herbal craft projects designed just for kids. While these are not herbal *recipes*, they are another opportunity for children to connect with the natural world while exploring their own creative gifts. From natural dyes to braided flower crowns, there are countless ways to engage in plant play!

Pocketknives and other sharp tools:

When foraging tender leaves, shoots, and blossoms, your hands are the only harvesting tools you'll need. For sturdier plants, however, a pair of strong scissors, branch cutters, or a pocketknife is a useful (even necessary) addition. If you are foraging with young children, decide for yourself when your child is ready to help with this task. You know your child better than anyone and can gauge when they are old enough to learn how to safely handle a knife. It is a skill that I encourage every parent to teach their child, and it will serve them for a lifetime.

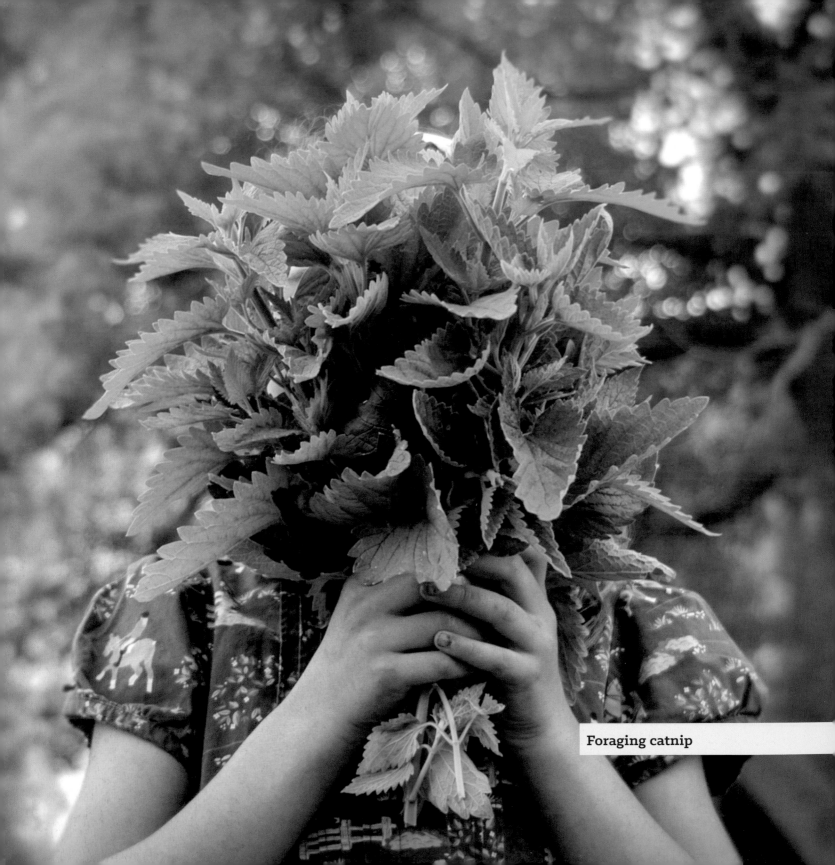

Foraging catnip

1 Getting Started

The world is full of useful plants—many of them rare, exotic, and obscure. This book, however, begins in the most familiar of places: your own backyard! In these pages, we'll explore ten common plants, some of which you may already know. These common backyard weeds form the backbone of kitchen herbalism. They are easy to find, easy to use, and have a variety of gifts to share with those who know how to use them.

In this chapter, we'll lay the foundation that every budding herbalist needs before diving in and working with the plants and recipes found later in the book.

Do you know a ray floret from a rhizome, or a leaflet from a lenticel? Don't fret! We'll explain these and other plant terms, and before you know it you'll be talking like a botanist. We'll also assemble our foraging and remedy-making tool kits and introduce the types of remedies you'll be crafting later in the book. And for those with an interest in foraging (picking your own herbs out in the wild), we'll lay out the basics for a fun, safe foraging outing so you can hit the trail and fill your basket with confidence.

Eat Your Weeds

What plants are growing in your backyard? I find that the plants that show up in our lives are often just what our bodies need. Identify the "weeds" that grow around your home, and then learn more about them. Even if you don't find the plants in this book in your neighborhood, learn about the wild plants that *are* abundant where you live. There might be edibles among them!

Some of the recipes in this book are for snacks, drinks, and other treats. Making "weeds" a part of your everyday diet might seem weird at first. But when you taste a dandelion fritter or add chickweed to your salad, you'll soon see why it's worth trying. Eating these wild plants is a simple way to get to know their flavors and the habitats and seasons in which they grow.

Of course, not all plants (or all plant parts) are safe to consume, so *always* do your homework before ingesting plants not listed as edible in the pages that follow. To do otherwise would be dangerous or even deadly.

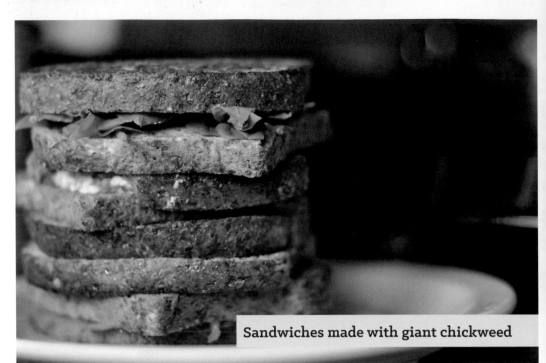

Sandwiches made with giant chickweed

Be Patient

Some herbs bring comfort and relief in a flash. Like a racing rabbit, they work fast and strong from the start to bring comfort in a hurry. A pinch of yarrow styptic powder on a cut, for example, stops bleeding and can reduce pain right away!

Other herbs are more like a tortoise, moving us slowly but steadily toward better health. These herbs won't seem to make a difference in the short term. But if you use them for a time, they can yield wonderful results. Think of these herbs like exercise or healthy eating. Make a habit of them, and your body will thank you!

Don't give up on these slow-but-steady tortoise recipes! Give them the time they need to generate positive changes. They are certainly worth the wait.

Follow Your Intuition

Making and using the recipes in this book is one part art, one part science, and one part intuition. Listen to your heart when selecting herbs and remedies for yourself and your family. If a plant is calling to you, learn about it. Do some research and find out what the herb has to offer and how to safely use it. Children often have a gift for this heart-led, instinctive understanding.

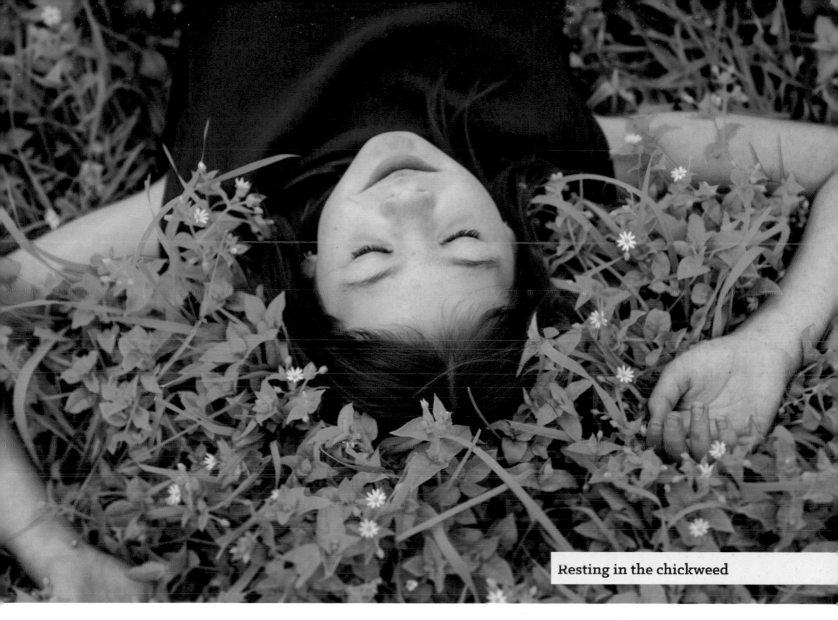

Resting in the chickweed

From my young daughter requesting pine needle tea when she had a cough to my teenage son asking if plantain was useful for earaches, they understand things they have never been taught. You have this same intuition!

Of course, our intuition cannot stand alone. It must always be followed by careful and thorough research to ensure safe use of our herbal friends. Nonetheless, it's a delightful place to begin.

Intuition is not just for plants that your body says "yes!" to. It's also for plants to which your body says "no!" Children in particular seem to know what their bodies need, a wisdom worth nurturing.

The Energy of Herbs

Warm, cool, damp, dry: these are some of the words herbalists use to describe the energetics of herbs and conditions.

If the notion of an herb being "cool" or "warm" seems a bit abstract, here's a little game to make it clear. Close your eyes and imagine sinking your teeth into a fresh, juicy cucumber. Cool? Damp? Indeed! Now imagine biting into a spicy chili pepper or chunk of raw gingerroot. So hot! While these are dramatic examples, this is the heart of herbal energetics.

People, too, tend toward warm or cool. We all know someone who always seems cold—wearing sweaters in summer and piling the bed with down blankets all year long. This is a cool

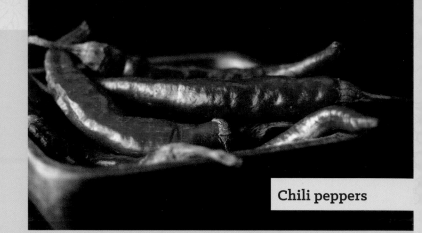

Chili peppers

constitution. Others are the opposite, favoring icy beverages and wearing short sleeves and sandals year-round. Being aware of our bodies can be helpful when choosing herbs to suit our specific needs.

Foraging

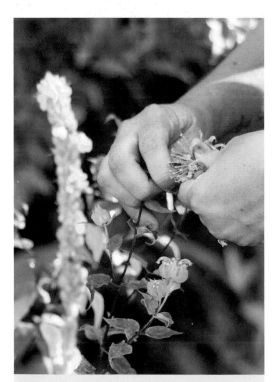

Foraging bee balm and mullein

While you can buy or plant the herbs in this book, foraging is a wonderful way to source them as well. If you want to try foraging, you can begin with a single, familiar plant, or set to work foraging all the species outlined in the following chapters. No need to go it alone . . . parents and kids make the best foraging teams!

For my kids and me, foraging is like a living treasure hunt. We find our baskets, pull on our boots, and then set out to see what is in season. Sometimes we come home with just what we were looking for, but most often, Mother Nature surprises us with treasures we never expected.

One of my favorite herbs to forage is nettle. After a long, cold winter, I can hardly wait to get outside in early spring and fill my basket with the deep-green shoots! I also love to pick wild peppermint, which grows in abundance near the creek at the edge of our farm. It's one plant I always smell before I see, adding an element of surprise to this never-planned-but-always-welcome excuse to forage.

When gathering herbs, always pick on a dry day, after the morning dew has evaporated. If it has been raining, wait to harvest until the leaves and flowers have dried completely. This will prevent your hard work from going

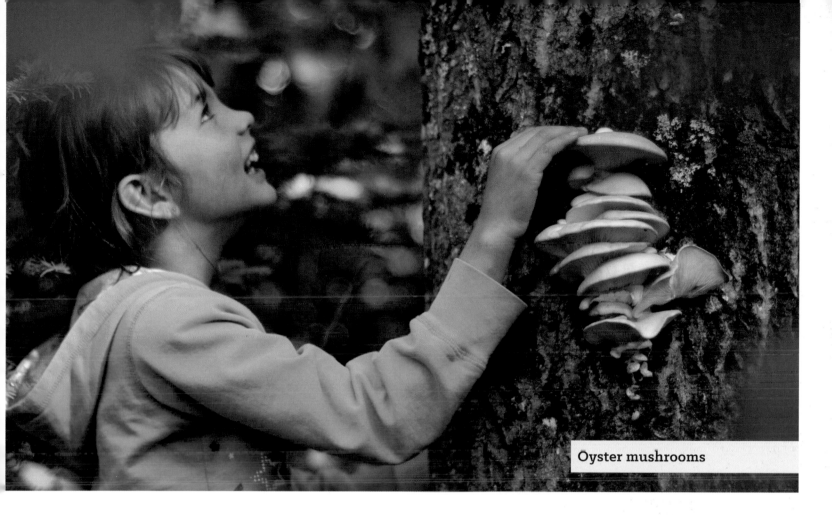

Oyster mushrooms

to waste, as wet herbs and flowers are quick to spoil.

Gather leaves in cloth shopping bags or tightly woven baskets. If desired, use plastic bags inside of your basket or tote to keep plants separated by species. Back home, empty your harvest on a table or countertop. Depending on what you picked, this may be messy work! You might need to work on a picnic table or outdoors on a deck or porch. Just be sure to be out of the wind if your plants are lightweight.

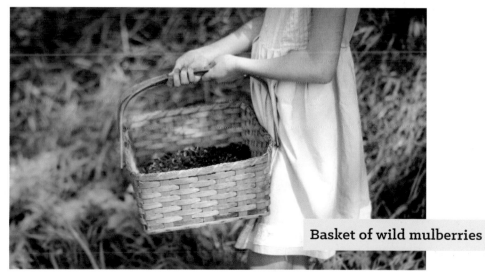

Basket of wild mulberries

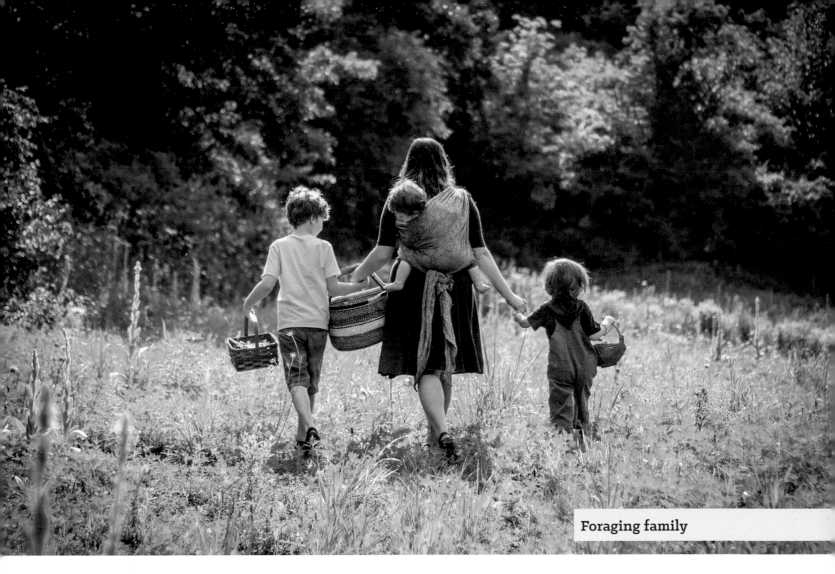

Foraging Basics

Ready to get started? Wait! There are a few things to know before you grab your basket and head for the woods. If you choose to forage some or all of the herbs for your recipes, always follow these simple guidelines to protect yourself, the plants, and the earth.

Be smart:

Prepare for your time in the woods before you head outside!

• Educate yourself before you set out to forage. Know how to positively identify the plants you are foraging and be absolutely certain of any dangerous lookalikes.

- Know your local toxic plants. Be on the lookout for poison ivy, poison oak, wild parsnip, and other potentially harmful plants found in your region.

- Wear appropriate clothing for your climate and apply mosquito and tick repellents and sun protection if needed. Throw a water bottle, raincoat, sweatshirt, and first aid kit in your bag . . . just in case.

Be safe:

Your safety is your first priority. Stay healthy by following the steps below.

- *Never* taste-test plants to determine their identity.

- Do not forage near busy roads; choose only plants growing a minimum of 50 feet from a roadway. Always harvest away from sprayed lawns and fields and areas that may contain pet waste.

- Never harvest a plant unless you are 100 percent certain of its identity.

- Always check with your adult if you have questions about the identity of a plant you have found.

Be respectful:

Respect landowners, plants, and the earth.

- Always get permission before you harvest from land that does not belong to you. The

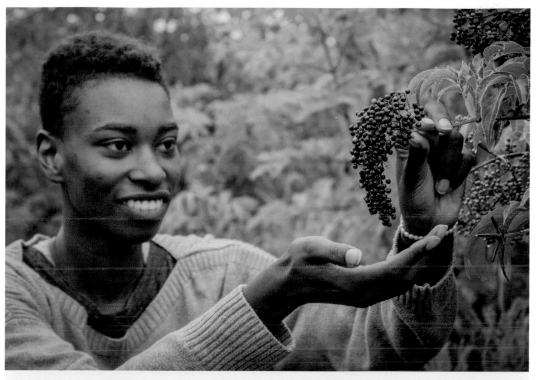

Foraging elderberries

question, "May I please pick some of your weeds?" is a fast way to make friends and share your love of wildcrafting with others.

- Follow the 10:1 rule. For every ten specimens of a plant you find, you are welcome to harvest one. This leaves plenty of flowers for the bees and food for wildlife, and ensures the plant can set seed for its continued survival. If you find

less than ten of any plant in an area, as tempting as it is, there aren't enough to pick. Check back again next season!

- Leave your foraging site better than you found it. Bag and toss any litter that you find while you are foraging. It's a small way of saying thank you to the fields and forests for all they provide.

"Leaflets three—let it be"

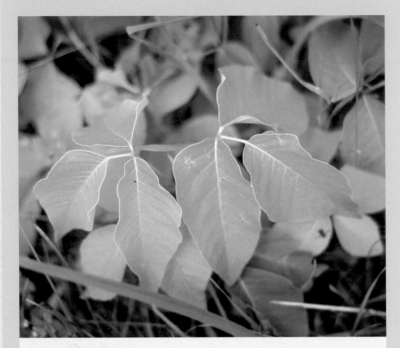

Poison ivy

The best protection against poison ivy (*Toxicodendron radicans*) is to simply stay on the lookout! Know how to identify poison ivy from a distance and keep your eyes open for it in the places where you explore.

Poison ivy is spread by contact with the oils found in the plant's leaves, stems, and roots. Contrary to popular belief, the fluid from a weeping sore does not spread the rash.

To identify poison ivy, look closely—but don't touch!

Never burn poison ivy. The troublesome oils become airborne and can cause serious, even life-threatening, health problems.

Habitat: Poison ivy is common in areas like roadsides, trailsides, parks, and campgrounds. In other words: places that people love to go!

Leaves: Each poison ivy leaf is composed of three leaflets. Leaf edges can be smooth or notched. Where the leaflets join together the stems are often red or pink, though not always. Leaves are attached alternately along the stem (though I don't encourage getting close enough to check). Leaves are usually shiny. In autumn, poison ivy turns scarlet red.

Stems: Poison ivy stems are thornless. While raspberries also have leaves comprised of three leaflets each, their stems bear thorns.

Growth habit: Poison ivy plants readily ramble and spread across the ground. If supported by tall grasses, brush, or trees, poison ivy is an accomplished climber as well, traveling high off the ground.

If you stumble into a patch of poison ivy, freeze and back out slowly the way you came in. To remove the oil from your skin, clean off as you would if you had motor oil or vegetable oil on your skin—by firmly wiping with a clean, dry cloth or paper towel. Never reuse the towel, as the oil will then spread to other parts of the body. Then wash skin well with soap and water, and dry with a clean towel. Wash clothing, tools, and shoes in hot water, being careful not to touch them with bare hands.

Foraging Tools

No special tools are needed to get started with foraging, but there are a few items that might help you in the field.

Harvest bags or baskets: A proper gathering bag is the key to an easy, relaxing harvest. Choose sturdy cotton shopping bags or, if you prefer, a tightly woven wicker basket. If desired, place a few plastic bags inside your basket or tote to keep plants from wilting on hot summer days.

Avoid gathering into plastic bags alone, as they tend to tear down the side. Also avoid any baskets with holes or gaps that may let plants fall out.

Shovel: A small trowel or, better yet, a sturdy garden shovel is a must for digging roots in the backyard, garden, and field. (Leave it at home if you're hiking, unless you're setting out specifically for roots.) Use your shovel for transplanting helpful "weeds" to more landscaping-friendly locations and for digging roots, such as burdock, ramps, or dandelions.

Sharp tools: A parent may need to assist you with branch cutters or a pocketknife. For example, pine and similar tree species may require a handheld pruner. However, most plants and this book can be harvested by hand, with at most a little help from a pair of scissors or a small knife.

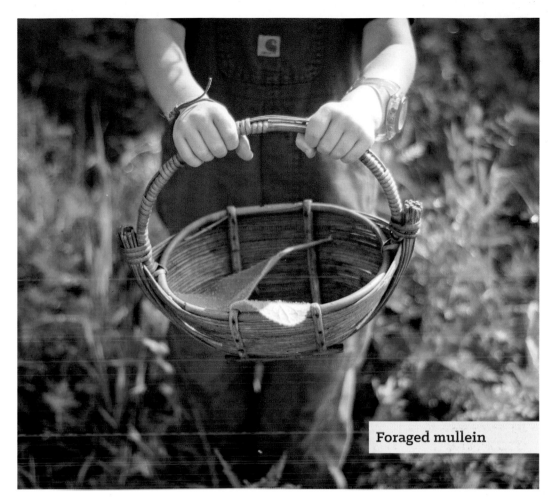

Foraged mullein

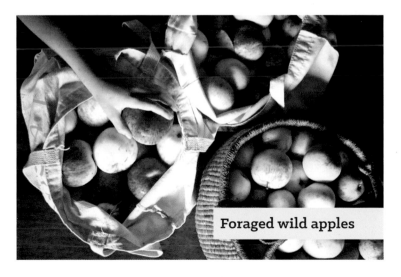

Foraged wild apples

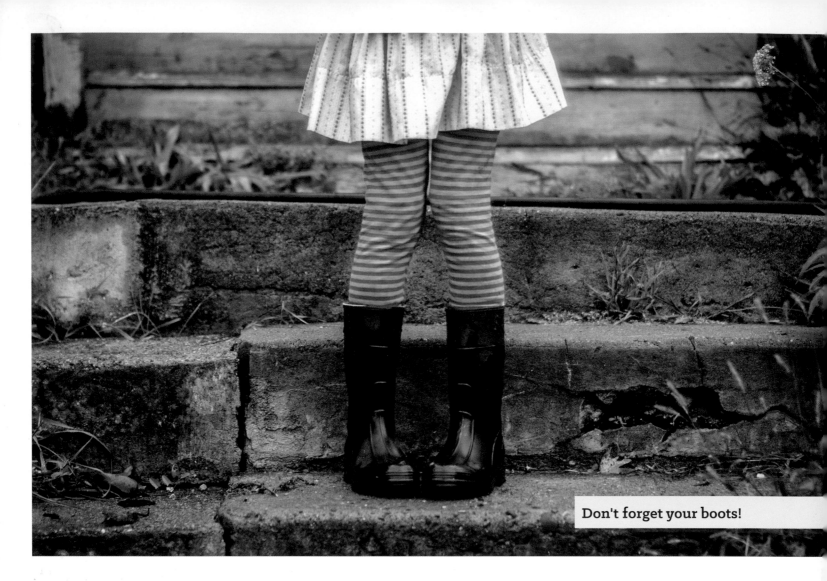

Don't forget your boots!

Protective clothing: If you're heading out for nettles, blackberries, or wild roses, protective clothing is a good idea! Choose sturdy fabrics to cover exposed skin and protect you from briars and brambles.

Closed-toed shoes: When you're out foraging it's wise to protect your feet. You'll likely go off the trail where poison ivy, stumps, brambles, and rocks await.

Garden gloves: When digging roots or harvesting nettle leaves, garden gloves are nice to have.

Insect repellent: If you live in a tick-prone region, apply natural insect repellent before you head out to the fields or forests (even in spring and fall, when the mosquitoes aren't out). You can also tuck in your shirt and tuck your pants into your socks to keep ticks out. Choose light-colored clothing and wear a hat to further protect yourself from biting insects.

Clean, Wilt, Dry, Garble, and Store

Once your basket is full of wild, foraged treasures, what's next? It's simple, really. Just follow these steps to prepare your herbs for use in the recipes later in the book!

Clean

Pick over your harvest, removing stray bits of grass, dirt, insects, and leaves that found their way in. Discard any wet or dirty leaves, keeping an eye out for bird droppings, cocoons, or insect eggs.

Wash roots thoroughly to remove soil and grit, and then rinse well under cold, running water. However, if you are foraging flowers or leaves to use for making remedies, do not wash your harvest! Washing introduces too much moisture and all but guarantees the spoilage of your harvest before it has a chance to be used.

When you are satisfied that your harvest is thoroughly picked over, it's time to wilt or dry your herbs!

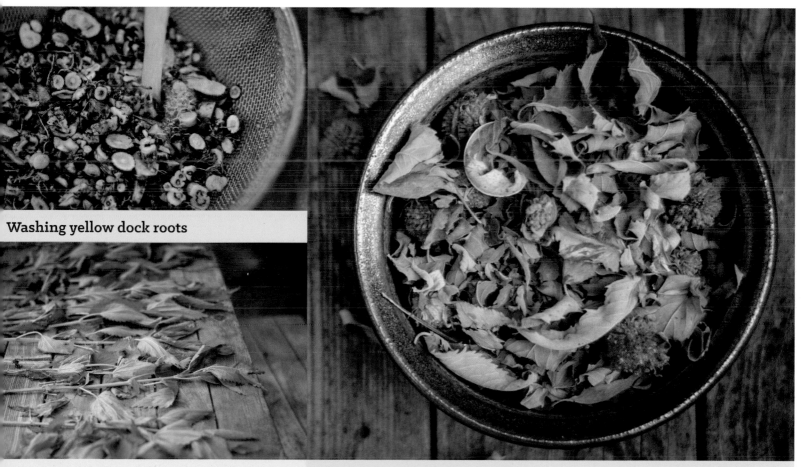

Washing yellow dock roots

Wilting nettle

Dried bee balm leaf and flower

Wilt

If you will be using your herbs fresh, you need to wilt the leaves and flowers. It's best to do this a day before proceeding with your recipe. Wilting removes excess moisture and extends the shelf life of your finished recipe.

To wilt, simply spread your plant out in a single layer, with little or no overlapping petals or leaves, on a cookie sheet, cooling rack, or table. Set everything in a shady spot to wilt (out of direct sunlight). Due to gusts of wind, it's best to wilt inside or on an enclosed porch.

Dry

Dried herbs can be stored for up to twelve months for use in teas, infusions, and decoctions. The plants must be first prepared by picking over for interlopers, such as pebbles and grass (as described on page 25). Roots can be washed well, patted dry, and then sliced or chopped.

The best method for drying herbs varies by climate. If you live in an area with warm, dry air, you can dry your herbs just like you would wilt them. Simply spread your plants out in a single layer on a cooling rack placed over a cookie sheet, and then place in an out-of-the way spot to dry. (If drying your herbs outside, be sure it is not a windy day, as you could lose your

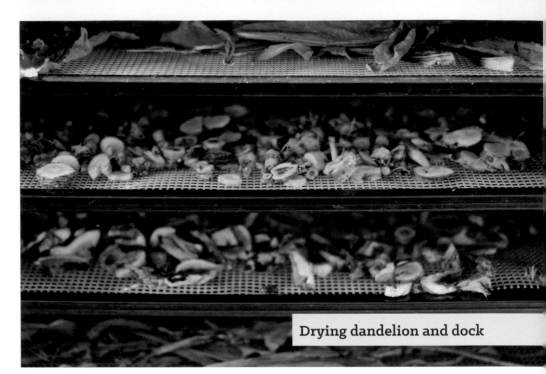

Drying dandelion and dock

harvest in a gust of wind!) How long your herbs take to dry depends both on the weather and on how moist your herbs were when harvested. Check them every few hours by pinching a leaf. When it crumbles easily between your fingers and thicker parts, such as stems or leaf veins, are also crisp, they're dry!

Herbs can also be tied into a brown paper bag and hung to dry, indoors or out. Fill the bag loosely with herbs, tie closed with kitchen twine, and hang until dry. Finally, herbs with long stems can be tied in small bundles and hung to dry from the rafters or a drying rack. Check them as described above to determine when they are thoroughly dry.

If you live in a humid or cool climate, lay your plants out in a single layer on a cooling rack over a cookie sheet. With the help of an adult, set the tray in an oven on very low heat (100–120°F). If possible crack your oven door open with a folded hot pad to allow moisture to escape and encourage drying. Dry herbs until crisp, without a hint of moisture left in the plants. Most herbs will be dry in four to twelve hours.

If you are lucky enough to own a dehydrator, by all means use that! These machines dry more herbs more quickly and evenly than an oven.

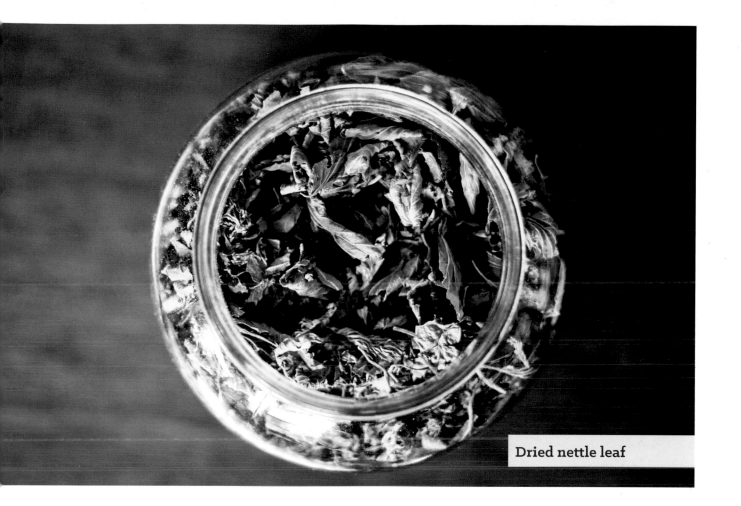

Dried nettle leaf

Some plants (those in the mint family, in particular) are quick to reabsorb moisture after drying. To ensure the quality of your harvest, put your herbs in jars as soon as possible after drying, and never store herbs that are not thoroughly dry. Discard any herbs that develop mold.

Garble

"Garble" is a funny word for a useful task: picking over our dried plants and separating the parts we want to keep from the parts we don't. We often garble to remove unwanted stems and seedheads.

Garbling is most easily done in a large, wide mixing bowl, providing room for more than one set of hands. It's a wonderful and satisfying job.

Store

Transfer your crisp, dried herbs to clean, dry mason jars. Lid your jars and label with the plant type and date of harvest. Do not label with sticky notes, as they easily drop off the jars. Use a permanent marker to make sure you can read your labels later in the year.

Store your jars of dried herbs in a dark cabinet or cupboard, away from heat and moisture. Dried herbs should be used within one year.

WHAT'S IN A NAME?

The common names of plants can differ by region, country, or culture. One plant could have ten or more of these nicknames! To further complicate things, names are sometimes shared between plants of different species. All of this can make discussing plants quite confusing.

Latin names to the rescue! These old-fashioned, scientific-sounding names are used by scientists, herbalists, and botanists. Each plant has one (and only one!) Latin name, and it is almost always in italics. We'll share them with you for the plants in the coming chapters. You don't need to use them when discussing plants, but it's handy to be familiar with them to clarify confusion when discussing plants with other herbal enthusiasts.

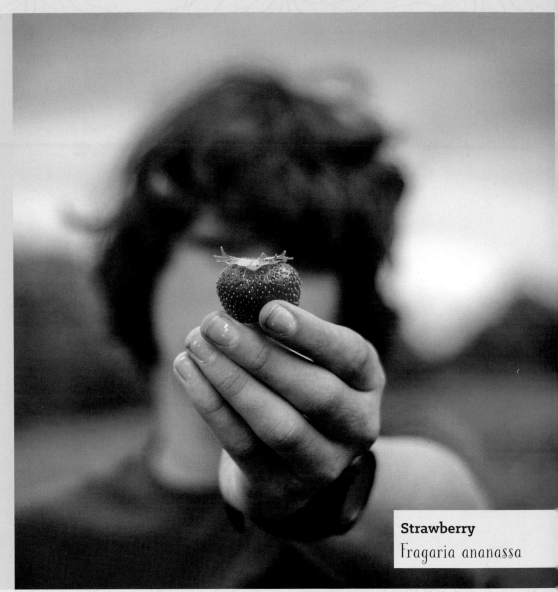

Strawberry
Fragaria ananassa

The Parts of Plants

In the vegetable garden, it's no surprise that different plants offer different useful parts. We harvest leaves (lettuce and cabbage), shoots and stalks (asparagus and rhubarb), roots (carrots and beets), fruits (tomatoes and strawberries), and more. And while some garden plants offer multiple edible parts (pea shoots and pea pods, or beet roots and beet greens, for example), others offer only one edible part.

It is much the same for herbs. Some plants offer fruit and flowers, others offer leaves and seeds, and others only roots or seeds or bark. What is useful varies by species, just as it does in the vegetable patch.

In the chapters that follow, we'll discover which parts of each plant are useful, focusing on leaves, flowers, fruits, seeds, bark, and roots. Pay attention to these plant parts and remember: just because one part of a plant is healthy and useful doesn't mean that all parts are! Just as eating the wrong part of a garden plant could make you very sick, the same is true for these plants. One of my favorite plants in this book, elderberry (*Sambucus nigra*), has edible berries and flowers. However, the leaves and branches are toxic if eaten.

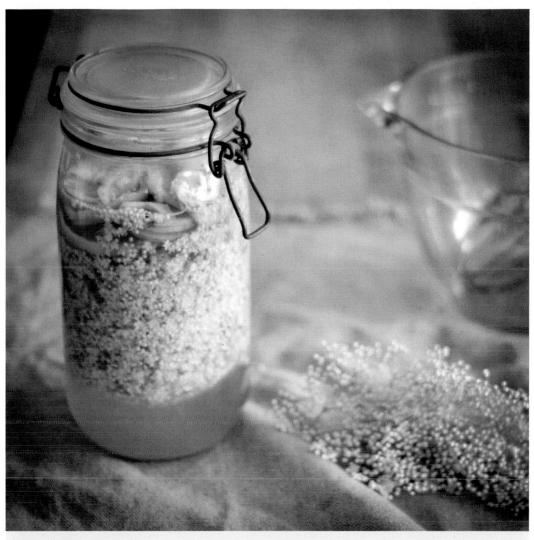

Elderflower infusion

NOTE: *Only use the plant parts recommended. And never substitute or experiment with parts you haven't thoroughly researched— it can be dangerous!*

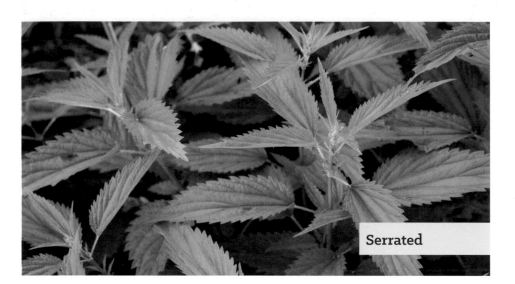

Serrated

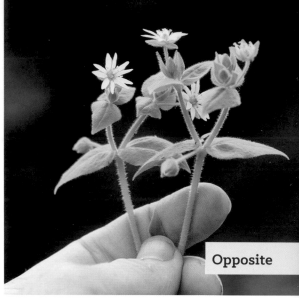

Opposite

Plant Terms to Know

The following terms will help transform you into a budding botanist. (They'll come up in the plant descriptions and recipes later in the book and are here for you to reference.)

Aerial parts: above-ground portions of a plant

Alternate: leaves arranged singularly along the stem, with one emerging on one side and another emerging on the other side farther up the branch

Basal rosette: a ring or whorl of leaves emerging directly from the ground

Biennial: a plant with a two-year life cycle, normally growing only leaves above ground the first year, and setting flowers the next

Composite: a member of the daisy family, featuring a compound flower head

Compound: made up of more than one part

> *NOTE: A compound leaf is comprised of several leaflets arranged along a single stem, versus a "simple" leaf, such as an oak or*

> *elm leaf, made of a single part. A compound flower is comprised of many smaller flowers clustered together in a single flower head.*

Disc florets: small, tubular florets lacking petals that form the central portion of most composite flowers

Distal: the far end of a branch or leaf

Fascicle: a bundle or cluster of needles, specific to pine species

Floret: a tiny flower that makes up a small part of a larger flower, as in a sunflower or dandelion

Herbaceous: lacking a hard, woody stem

Leaflet: a small leaf-like structure that forms a part of a compound leaf

Lenticels: raised pores found on the stem of a woody plant, which act as "breathing" ports and allow for the exchange of gases between the plant and the atmosphere

Midrib: a sturdy vein running down the center of a leaf

Opposite: leaves arranged in pairs along the stem

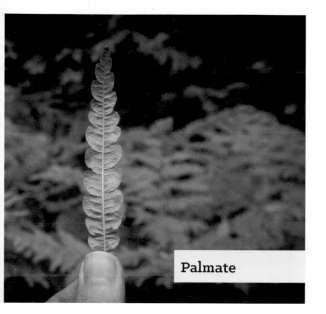

Palmate

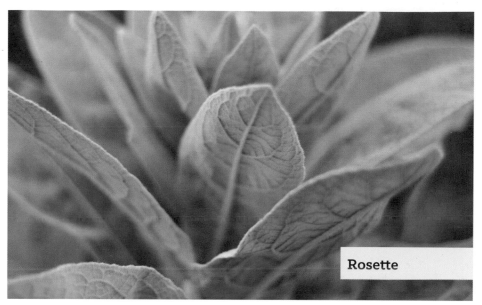

Rosette

Palmate: a lobed leaf with midribs that all radiate from one point, like fingers radiating out of a palm

Pinnate: a lobed leaf with leaflets or lobes arranged on the stem in pairs along a central midrib

Pistil: the female organs of a flower, from which seeds develop

Pith: a soft, spongy, normally tan or white tissue found inside the stems of some species

Ray florets: small florets normally bearing a single elongated petal each that comprise the outer ring of many composite flowers (daisy and sunflower, for example)

> **NOTE:** *Some species bear flowers comprised entirely of ray florets.*

Rhizomes: roots that spread horizontally under the surface of the soil, often sending up shoots at intervals along its length

Rosette: a cluster of over-lapping leaves arranged in a rose-like fashion, often found growing directly on the ground

Serrated: toothed or jagged edge

Stamen: the male organ of a flower, from which pollen arises

Stem: the main part or body of a plant, emerging from the roots and bearing the other plant parts (leaves, branches, etc.)

Taproot: a long, relatively straight main root growing downward into the earth from a plant

Umbel: an umbrella-shaped cluster of flowers or berries

Types of Plant Remedies

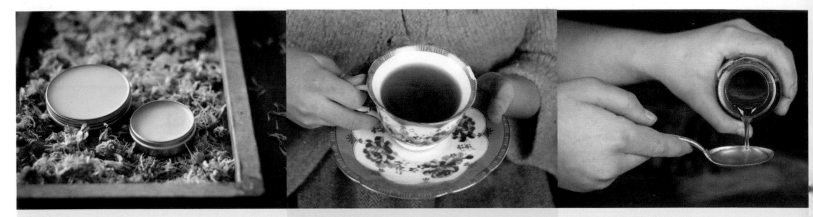

Calendula salve   **Peppermint tea**   **White pine syrup**

Many herbal remedies are simply plant-based treatments for injury or illness. Making a remedy can be as simple as chewing up a fresh leaf and putting the resulting green mash onto a bee sting. (Really! We'll make some later on in the book.) But remedies can also be much more elegant and complex than that.

Also, keep in mind that most recipes in the chapters that follow can be varied to your liking. Change them to suit your taste or the herbs you have available. If you find that an infused vinegar is hard for you to swallow, add honey and enjoy it as an oxymel (vinegar-honey syrup) instead. These are *your* recipes after all. You can use them exactly as written or customize to your heart's content! The choice is up to you. Here are some remedies we will explore.

Poultice: Mashed herbs applied directly to the skin—either chewed or crushed with a mortar and pestle—are called a poultice. A poultice allows the herbal juices to go to work directly on the problem area. While they aren't pretty, they are quick, effective, and easy to make.

Infusion: If you've ever made a cup of tea, you've made an infusion. Infusions are herbs steeped in water, oil, or vinegar, which are then either drunk or applied to the skin. Infusion times vary widely, depending on what you're making. It can be as little as a few minutes for an herbal tea, to overnight for a strong herbal infusion, or as long as several weeks or even months for an infused oil.

Decoction: A decoction is similar to an infusion, but made of the sturdier parts of a plant, such as seeds, bark, and roots. Extraction takes longer for these more stubborn plant materials, so we normally simmer a decoction until the liquid is reduced by half.

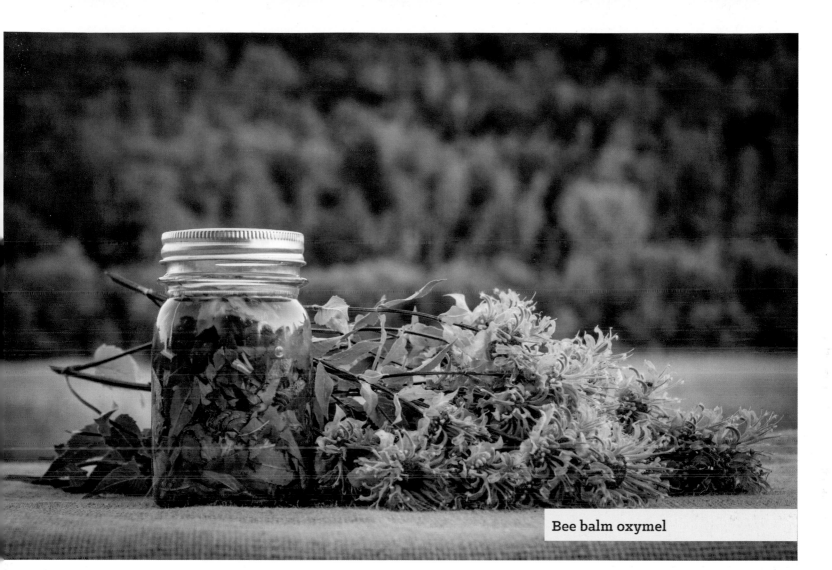

Bee balm oxymel

Syrup: Syrups are easy to make and delicious to take! They are crafted from either honey and fresh herbs or honey and a decoction of dried herbs in water. Syrups can be enjoyed in teas, on pancakes, or straight off of the spoon, depending on the herbs and intended uses.

Glycerite: Made with glycerin and water, glycerites are sweet, mild formulas that are especially suited for kids.

Oxymel: Oxymels are made with a combination of raw apple cider vinegar and honey. They can be quite delicious on their own and they make a fine base for salad dressings as well.

Salve: Herbal salves (also called balms) are made from herb-infused oils. By simply adding beeswax to the strained oil, a smooth, easy-to-use balm results.

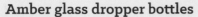
Amber glass dropper bottles

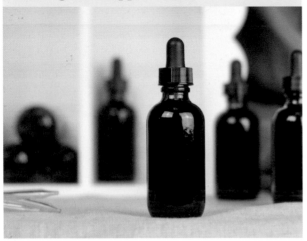

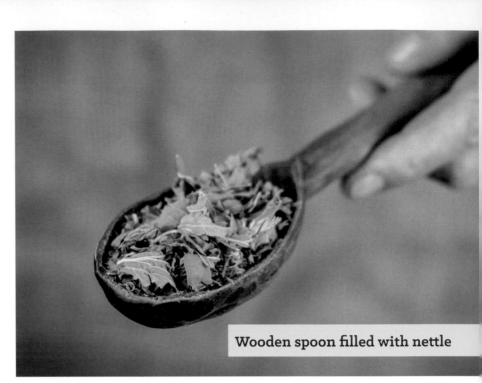
Wooden spoon filled with nettle

Useful Tools and Equipment for Remedies

Stainless steel pots: "Non-reactive" pots or pans (not made of aluminum or cast iron and without a nonstick coating) are required for any stovetop remedy making. If you don't have stainless steel, glass or unchipped enamel pots are good choices as well.

Steel or wooden spoons: Use a stainless steel spoon, or a wooden spoon you don't mind staining, when stirring these recipes. Avoid using plastic, as it may leach chemicals.

Measuring cups and spoons: Again, stainless steel or glass are best, but use what you have. Plastic tools may be discolored by some ingredients.

Glass jars: Mason jars are very useful and we'll rely on them in many recipes. If you don't already have a stash of glass jars in the basement or pantry, they are easy to find second-hand or at your local grocery, hardware, or department store. If you are reusing jam, nut butter, or pickle jars, make sure that they are completely clean and free of odors and have a tight-fitting lid. Stock up on a variety of sizes from quarter-pint to quart for the recipes that follow.

Glass dropper bottles: Glass dropper bottles are nice for storing some of the recipes in this book, although they aren't necessary. If you would like to use dropper bottles for your finished formulas, you can purchase them at some natural foods stores, or online through the sources listed in the resources section (see page 171).

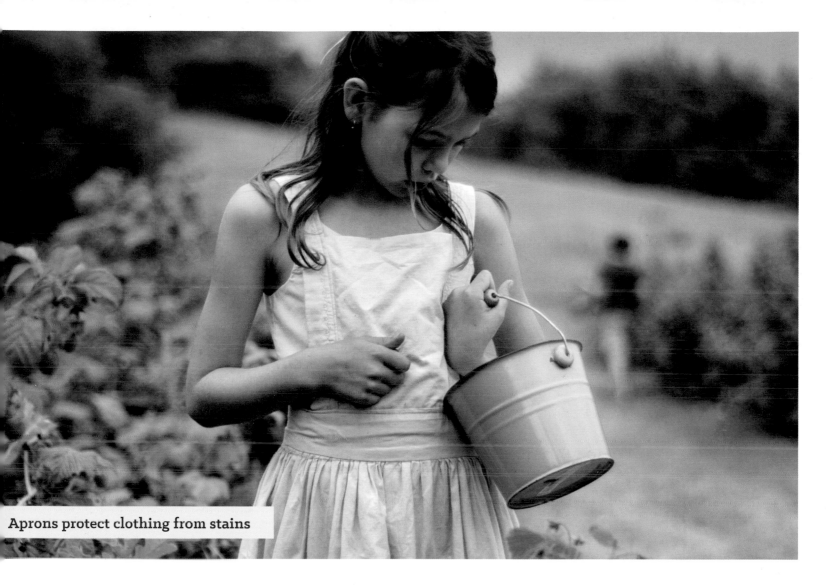

Aprons protect clothing from stains

Choose amber or cobalt if possible, as these dark bottles are better at keeping sunlight out than clear bottles and extend the useful life of your remedies.

Plastic or nonreactive lids: Many of these recipes require a plastic or other non-metal lid. If you don't have a plastic lid, you can line a regular mason jar lid with waxed paper, parchment, or a plastic sandwich bag instead.

Glass measuring pitcher: A glass or steel measuring pitcher is useful for pouring balms and oils. They come in a variety of sizes, but a two-cup measure will work for most of these recipes.

Apron: When you are working with oils and herbs, an apron will keep you clean! Protect your clothes by donning one before you get to work.

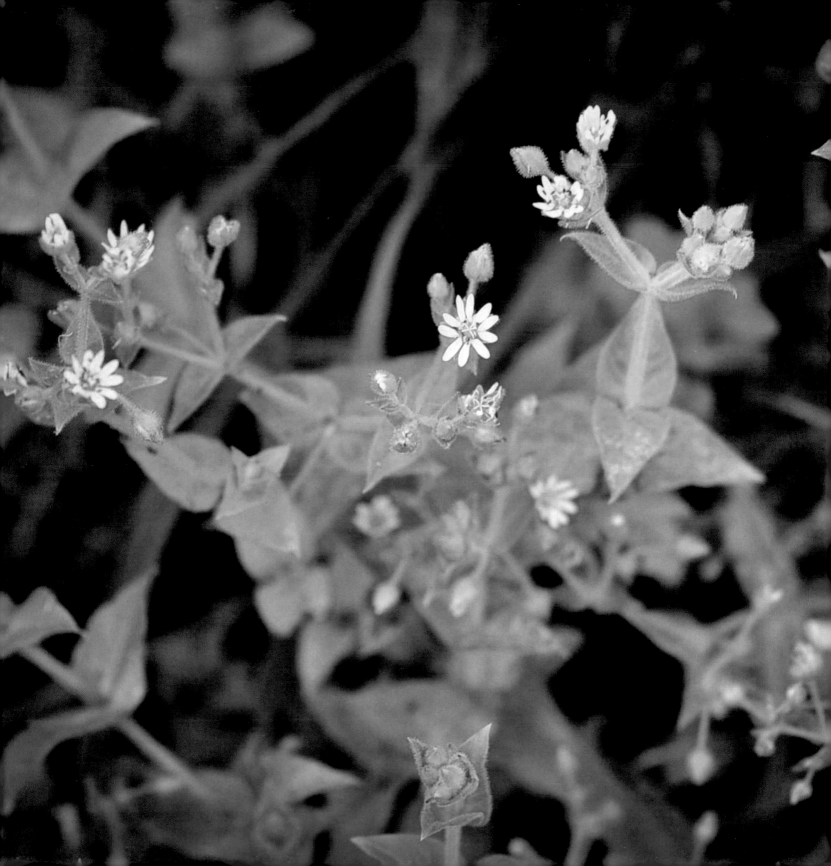

2 Chickweed

Oh, hello . . . it's lovely to meet you. My name is Chickweed. I've been here at the edge of the garden for ever so long. Perhaps you overlooked me—many people do. It's to be expected. I like to stay close to the ground, which makes me easy to miss. Take a closer look and you'll discover that, despite appearing small, I'm actually quite tall. I just prefer life close to the earth where things are cool and moist, just like me.

My Latin name, *Stellaria*, means "little star" and hints at the shape of my small white flowers. If you count my petals, you might be surprised to find that there are only five on each flower, but at first glance most people think there are ten. Each petal is so deeply lobed that it looks like two.

There are many gifts that I'm happy to share with those who befriend me.

I can calm a hot, itchy rash, comfort cuts and scrapes, and soothe red, dry, or itchy eyes. As a cooling herb, I'm a delightful snack on a summer day. I also help the body take up nutrition from other foods. So please don't think of me as a weed! On the contrary: I am a nourishing food and a soothing remedy. I have so much to offer those who choose to be my friend.

Latin Name:

Stellaria species

Parts Used:
leaves, flowers, and stems (all the above-ground parts)

Energetics:
cool and moist

Chickweed is a helpful herb for:
- Cooling the body, both inside and out
- Calming hot or itchy rashes
- Soothing irritated eyes
- Quieting stomach upset and easing constipation
- Nourishing the body with vitamins and minerals
- Aiding nutrient uptake

Field Identification

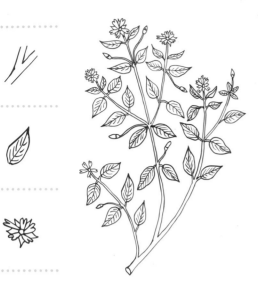

To identify chickweed in the field, look for its key distinguishing characteristics. Use the photograph on the right as a guide. Note: There are several different species of chickweed found throughout the United States and Europe. While all *Stellaria* species are useful externally, we will focus on the larger, more succulent varieties, since we will be using chickweed for food as well as for remedies. These species include both giant chickweed (*Stellaria aquatica*) and common chickweed (*Stellaria media*), pictured below. Both of these species are well-suited for the recipes in this chapter. If you have a different kind of chickweed, by all means give it a try!

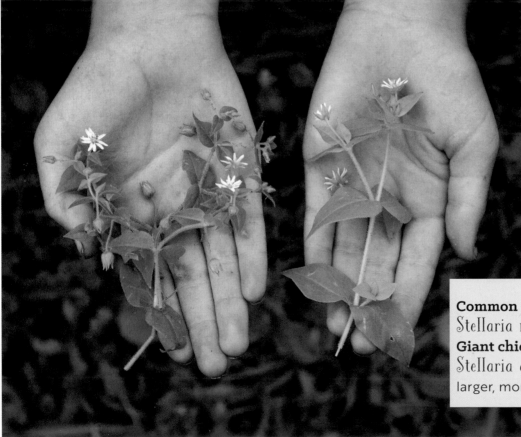

Common chickweed
Stellaria media, shown at left, and
Giant chickweed
Stellaria aquatica, shown at right. Notice the larger, more succulent leaves of giant chickweed.

Stem:

Chickweed stems ramble along the ground in a tangled mat. Each stem grows from 4 to 16 inches long in a zigzagging fashion. Look closely, and you'll see lines of tiny, white hairs and swollen joints between stem sections. The stem is juicy and snaps enthusiastically when harvested, almost as if a fine elastic thread is running through it.

Leaves:

Chickweed leaves are arranged oppositely (in matched pairs) along the succulent stem. Leaves growing toward the bottom of the plant tend to have a short stalk (leaf-stem), while leaves toward the tip are stalkless, with the leaf base partially encircling the stem. Leaves are tender and juicy. The tops of chickweed leaves are smooth, while the undersides are often covered with a fine coating of tiny, white hairs.

Flowers:

At first glance, chickweed flowers appear to have ten petals each. A closer inspection, however, reveals just five petals per flower. Each petal is deeply lobed, cleaving the petal nearly in two. Flower buds are fuzzy and, like the underside the leaves, covered in fine, white hairs.

Growth:

Chickweed tends to grow in a tangle of sprawling stems, rambling across the ground. Though each stalk can grow over a foot long, they only grow upright when supported by surrounding grasses and herbs. Chickweed stems are branching and the roots are shallow.

Range:

Chickweed is native to Europe and found throughout much of North America.

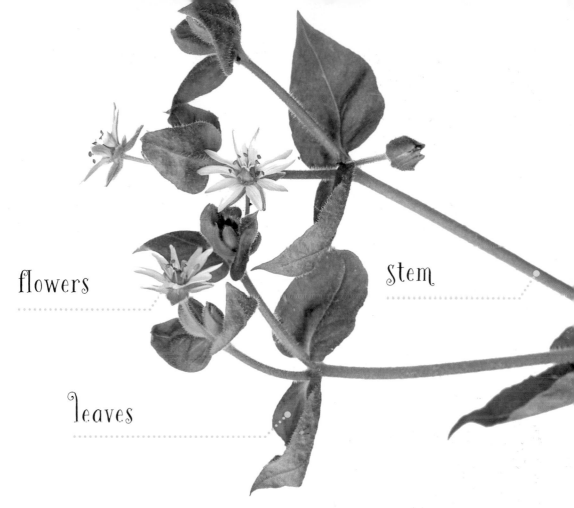

flowers

leaves

stem

Habitat:

Chickweed prefers moist, shady areas. Look for it on the darker, northern side of buildings and sheds, under shrubs, in forests, and along sheltered stream banks. It is also a common garden weed, so you might find it under your tomatoes or green beans!

Lookalikes:

Scarlet pimpernel resembles chickweed and is not safe to eat! However, with a little attention to detail, the two are easy to tell apart.

Scarlet pimpernel has smooth, hairless stems, as opposed to the rows of fine, white hairs that appear on chickweed stems.

When in bloom, scarlet pimpernel flowers range from orange to red to blue and are composed of five unlobed petals. Chickweed flowers each contain five deeply lobed petals (looking like ten tiny petals) and are *always* white.

Fresh Chickweed Spit Poultice

INGREDIENTS

❊ 1 or 2 sprigs of fresh chickweed

Tumbles, scrapes, and skinned knees happen. But fear not! An herbal poultice is ready to help, even when your first aid kit isn't close at hand. Think of a poultice as a gooey green bandage from Mother Nature's first aid kit. A smear of mashed chickweed might not be pretty, but it quickly reduces pain, cools hot rashes, and stops bleeding. What a comfort to have when you need it most!

TIME: Less than 1 minute, not including foraging time | **YIELD:** 1 teaspoon

Instructions

1. Pick a handful of fresh, healthy chickweed. (Be sure you harvest from a place free of pets and lawn chemicals, and away from busy roads.)

2. Double-check that your chickweed is free of debris and dirt, rinse with fresh water if desired, and then pop the sprigs into your mouth.

3. Chew until the chickweed becomes a thick, green paste. Since most people think chickweed is delicious, this step is easy.

4. Slather the paste onto cuts, scrapes, bee stings or rashes. Gross, I know, but it's effective!

Variation: The Spit-Free Spit Poultice

If the idea of putting on a remedy that has been chewed up and spit out is too much for you, don't fret. You can still benefit from a fresh herbal poultice, sans saliva. The method you use is entirely up to you! For the record, we think the first version is more fun, simple, and effective. (Unless, of course, you're squeamish!)

Instructions

1. Pick a handful of fresh, healthy chickweed. As mentioned before, make sure you harvest from a place free of pets and lawn chemicals, and away from busy roads.

2. Double-check that your chickweed is free of debris and dirt, rinse with fresh water, and then coarsely chop with a kitchen knife.

3. Grind up the chickweed with a mortar and pestle or in a food processor with a drop or two of water.

4. Apply as described above.

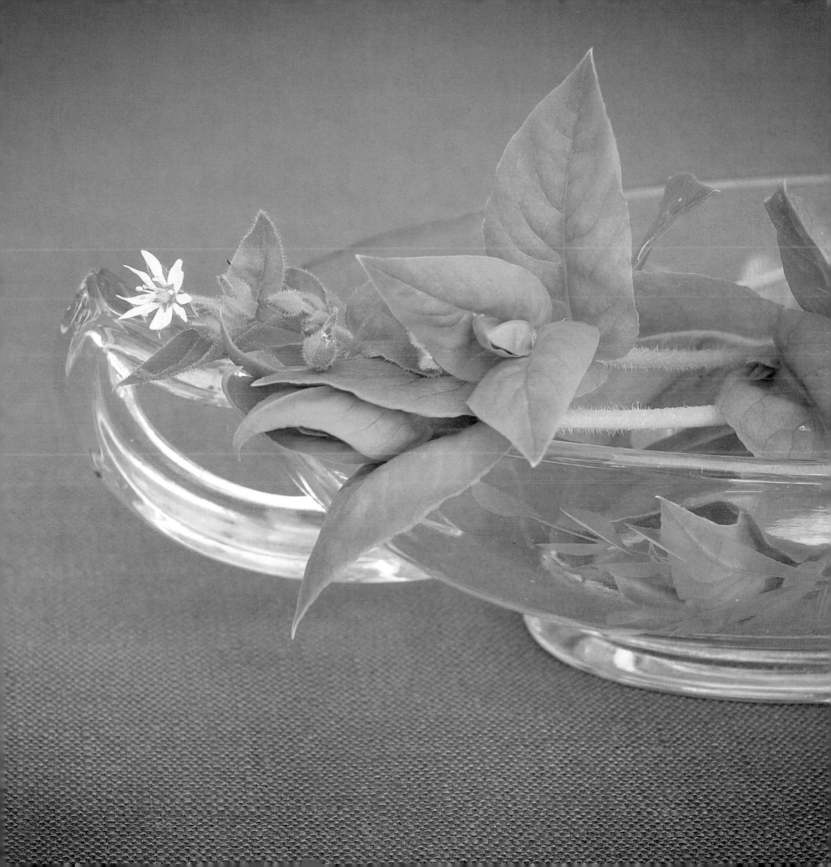

Chickweed Salad

INGREDIENTS

Salad

- ❋ 2 to 4 cups fresh chickweed leaves and tips
- ❋ 4 to 6 cups baby greens, or lettuce of your choice
- ❋ A handful of edible flowers, such as violet, chive, nasturtium, or dandelion, if desired

Lemon Vinaigrette Salad Dressing

- ❋ ¼ cup olive oil
- ❋ 1 tablespoon raw apple cider vinegar
- ❋ Zest of 1 lemon
- ❋ 2 tablespoons freshly squeezed lemon juice
- ❋ 1 tablespoon raw honey
- ❋ 1 garlic clove, finely minced or crushed
- ❋ ½ teaspoon prepared yellow or brown mustard
- ❋ Pinch of salt
- ❋ A few grinds of black pepper

Most people agree: foraged chickweed is delicious! This salad uses wild chickweed to add interest to otherwise tame greens. It's an easy way to get started with foraged foods, and you can gradually increase the chickweed as your family gets used to the idea of eating foraged fare. The salad and dressing can be prepared a day in advance and stored separately until ready to serve.

TIME: 15 minutes or less, not including foraging time | **YIELD:** 6 servings

Instructions

1. Pick over the chickweed and remove any garden debris. Pull the leaves off of any long stem segments and separate the tender tips just below the second pair of leaves. Discard all long stem segments.

2. Tear the lettuce into bite-sized pieces, and then wash the lettuce and chickweed and spin dry.

3. Toss the greens in a salad bowl and sprinkle with edible flowers, if you're using them.

4. Place the dressing ingredients in a half-pint mason jar. Cover the jar with a tight-fitting lid and shake well to combine. Alternately, you can blend all the ingredients with a whisk in a medium-sized bowl until well combined.

5. Serve the salad and pass the dressing at the table. Enjoy!

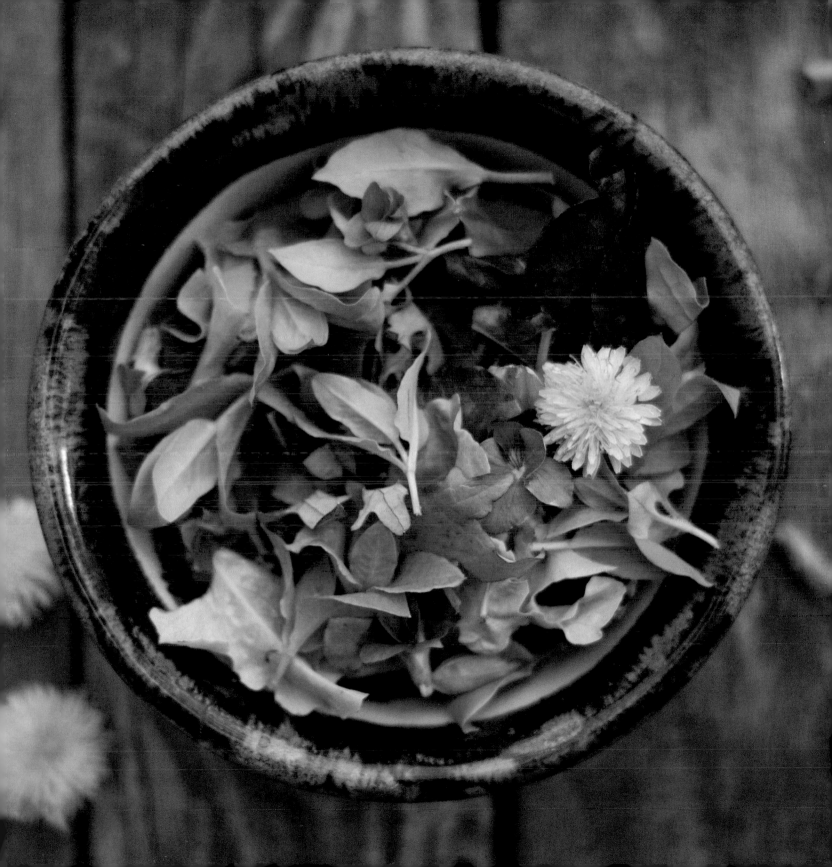

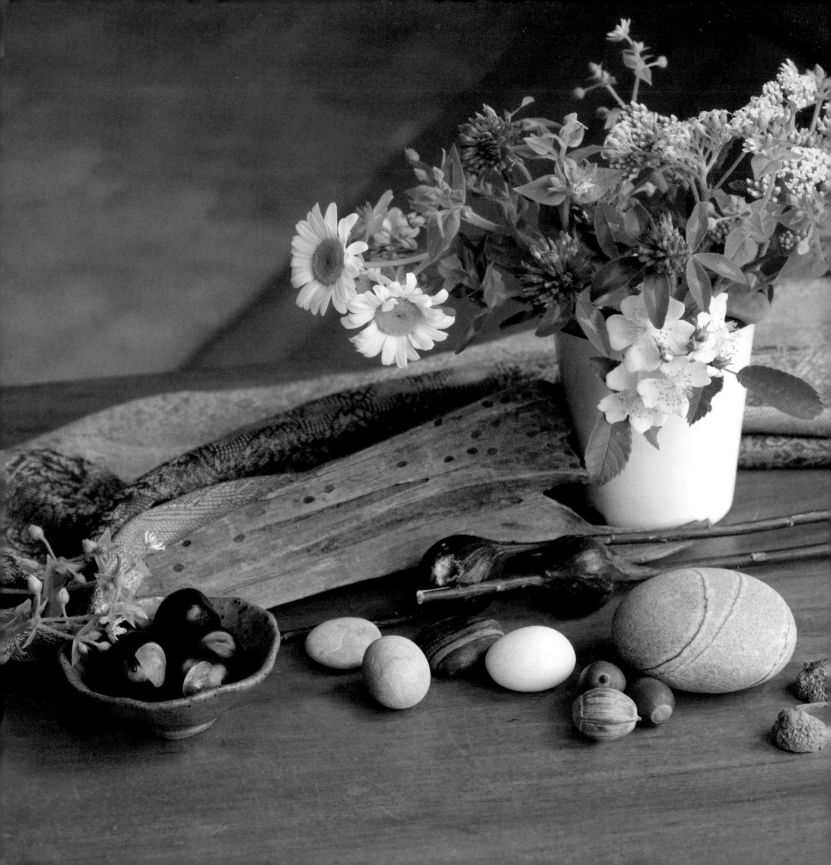

Nature Corner

There's no need to leave nature behind when you come inside at the end of the day! Create a seasonal nature corner and keep a bit of the natural world close at hand indoors. This out-of-the-way display is just the place to showcase your ever-changing collection of treasures and will keep you inspired for your next adventure to the forest.

Supplies

There are no hard-and-fast rules about what to use in your nature corner—only that you follow your inspiration! Rather than a play place, think of your nature corner as a quiet space to study and connect with the natural world. (For this reason, nature corners are best set up out of reach of toddler-aged children.)

Include seasonal items that you find outside, such as:

- Acorns, pine cones, seedpods, and tree bark
- Dried leaves
- Seashells
- Rocks and crystals
- Fresh or dried wildflowers, grasses, and herbs
- Driftwood, tree branch, or other piece of interesting wood

Add items that conjure the season, such as:

- A cloth to drape over the table in a seasonally appropriate color (e.g. soft green for spring, deep green for summer, brown for autumn, and white for winter)
- A bouquet of seasonal flowers from the market or your garden
- A pot of sprouted wheatgrass
- Pine boughs
- Forced flowering branches from a flowering tree
- Small felt or wooden figurines of humans or other animals (e.g. rabbits in spring, foxes in summer, deer in winter, etc.)
- Handmade or craft-store bird's nests (polished stones make convincing eggs!)

Instructions

1. Choose an out-of-the-way corner of your home in which to set up your nature space. A windowsill, shelf, or dresser top will do nicely.

2. Drape the shelf with a cloth and add a manageable branch or piece of driftwood to form your foundation.

3. As you explore the natural world, add the treasures that you bring home in your pockets and hands.

4. Keep your nature corner fresh by discarding items that have faded or that you have lost interest in and replacing them with new finds.

5. As the season changes, switch out your cloth for one that suits the world outside.

A NOTE ON FEATHERS AND NESTS: Feathers and nests are tempting, beautiful nature finds. However, these items from most bird species are protected by federal law in the United States. These treasures should be enjoyed outside and left where they are. The exception is feathers from pigeons, European starlings, and English house sparrows, as well as pheasant, wild turkey, grouse, and partridge, with a permit. Additional details can be found in the Migratory Bird Treaty Act.

Chickweed Pesto

Traditional Italian pesto, a flavorful sauce made of basil and garlic, is a staple in our home. We love to experiment with herbal pesto variations, such as watercress, wild ramps, and even nettle leaf. In this herbal version we're adding plenty of succulent chickweed. The mild flavor is delicious on pizza, pasta, or even sandwiches.

TIME: Less than 15 minutes, not including foraging time | **YIELD:** 1½ cups

INGREDIENTS

- ¼ cup pine nuts or walnuts
- 2 cups chickweed leaves and tips
- ½ cup basil
- ¾ cup olive oil
- 2 large cloves garlic, smashed or coarsely chopped
- ⅛ teaspoon salt

Instructions

1. Toast the nuts in a dry skillet over medium heat. Stir constantly and remove from the heat when they have begun to brown and smell fragrant. Set aside to cool.

2. Pick over the chickweed and remove any debris. Pull the leaves off of any long stem segments and separate the tender tips just below the second pair of leaves from the top. Discard all long stems.

3. Combine the nuts and chickweed with the remaining ingredients in a food processor. Process until fairly smooth, shutting off your machine and scraping the sides of the bowl frequently.

4. When your pesto is fairly smooth and no large leaves or nuts remain, taste and add additional salt if desired.

To use

Spread on grilled cheese sandwiches or homemade pizza, or use as a dip for grilled chicken. My family even loves it served on scrambled eggs!

Storage

This pesto will keep for 5 to 7 days, covered in the refrigerator. For longer storage, place heaping tablespoon-sized scoops of pesto onto a cookie sheet. Place the filled tray in the freezer. (You can also freeze pesto in an ice cube tray.) When the pesto is frozen, remove it from the tray with a thin spatula and transfer to a storage container. Label and freeze the pesto for up to one year. When you're ready to use it, remove and thaw as many pesto pucks as you desire.

Variation: Chickweed Pesto with Wild Ramps or Cilantro

Substitute a handful of wild ramps or garlic scapes for garlic cloves, or try cilantro in place of the basil.

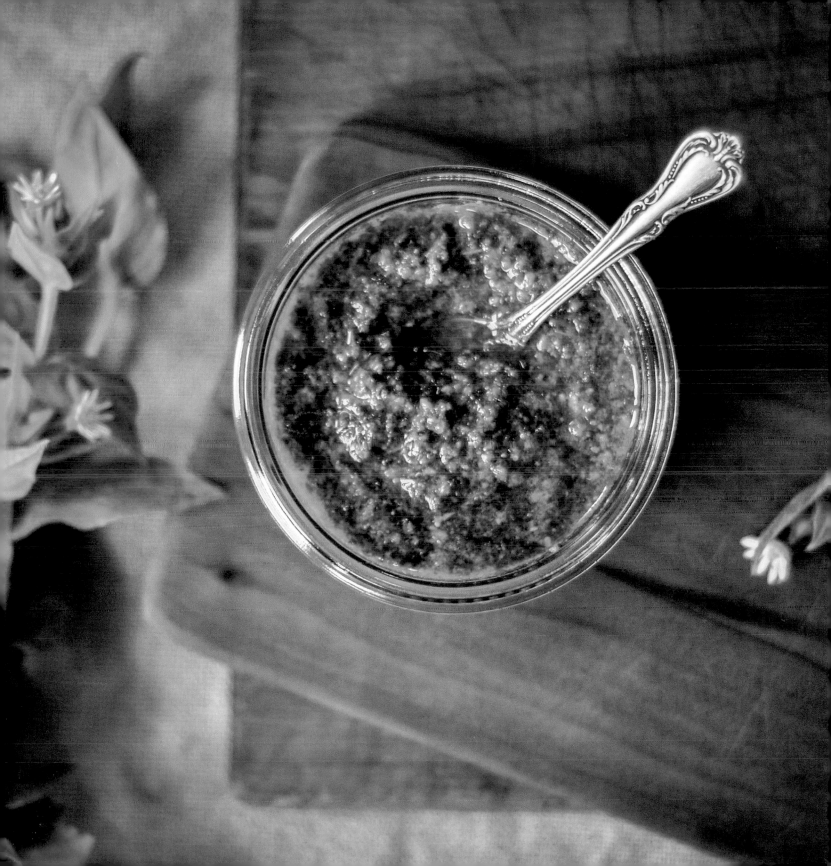

Itch-Fix Balm

NOTE: We will make this balm in two steps: first we will infuse the oil with the chickweed; then we will use our infused oil to craft our balm.

Don't let that itchy rash drive you wild! Just a dab of Itch-Fix Balm and you'll be feeling like yourself in no time. Apply it on bug bites, poison ivy rashes, eczema, and itchy, peeling sunburns. Aaaah . . . relief!

STEP 1: INFUSE YOUR OIL

ACTIVE TIME: Less than 1 hour, not including foraging and wilting or drying time
TOTAL TIME: 24 hours or 3 to 4 weeks, depending on method | **YIELD:** 5 ounces

INFUSING OIL

- ½ cup fresh, wilted, chopped chickweed, or scant ¼ cup dried
- 1 cup organic olive oil

Instructions

1. Infused oils are among the easiest plant remedies to make. Using the ingredients listed at left, follow the instructions on pages 169 or 170 to create yours. Choose whichever method you prefer: solar or stovetop.

STEP 2: MAKE YOUR BALMS

After your oil is infused and strained, it's time to create your balms!

ACTIVE TIME: Less than 30 minutes | **TOTAL TIME:** 1 hour

MAKING BALM

- ½ cup chickweed-infused oil
- 1 tablespoon plus 1 teaspoon grated beeswax
- 12 drops peppermint essential oil (optional)
- 6 drops lavender essential oil (optional)

Instructions

1. Combine the chickweed-infused oil and beeswax in a small stainless steel or glass pan.

2. Warm the mixture over very low heat until the beeswax has melted.

3. Remove the pot from the heat, let the mixture cool for 1 to 2 minutes, and then add the essential oils, if using. Gently swirl or stir to combine.

4. Carefully pour the mixture into small glass jars or metal tins. If the balm hardens during pouring, simply rewarm over very low heat.

5. Allow the balms to sit undisturbed until cool, and then lid and label.

To use

Apply liberally as needed to itchy rashes and irritated skin. Avoid the eyes and eye area.

Storage

Stored in a cool, dry place, Itch-Fix Balm should last for up to 1 year.

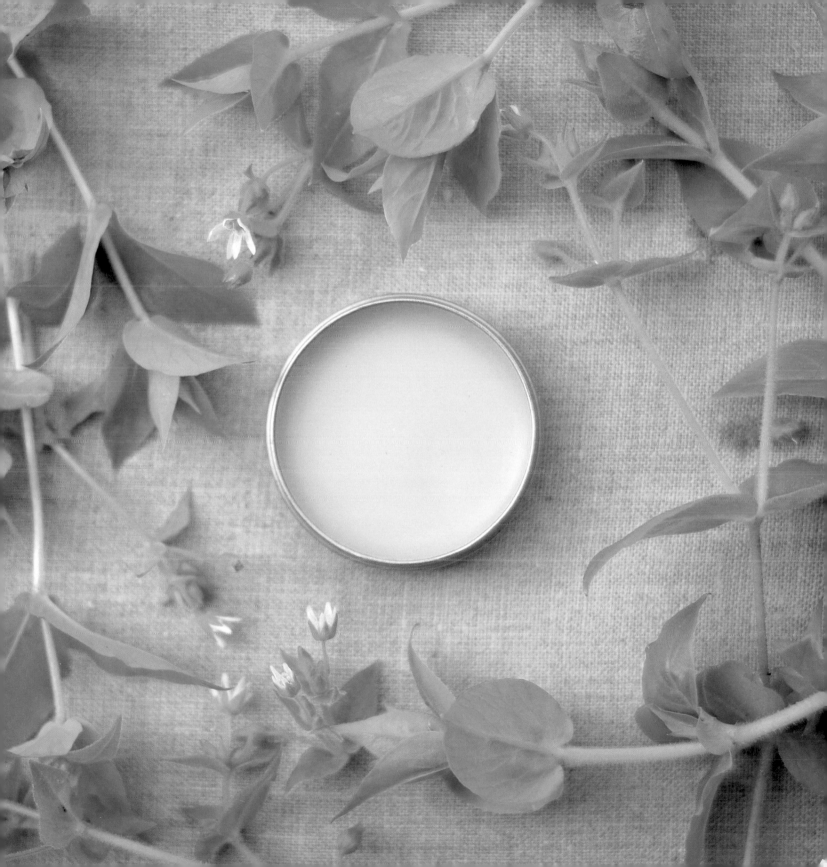

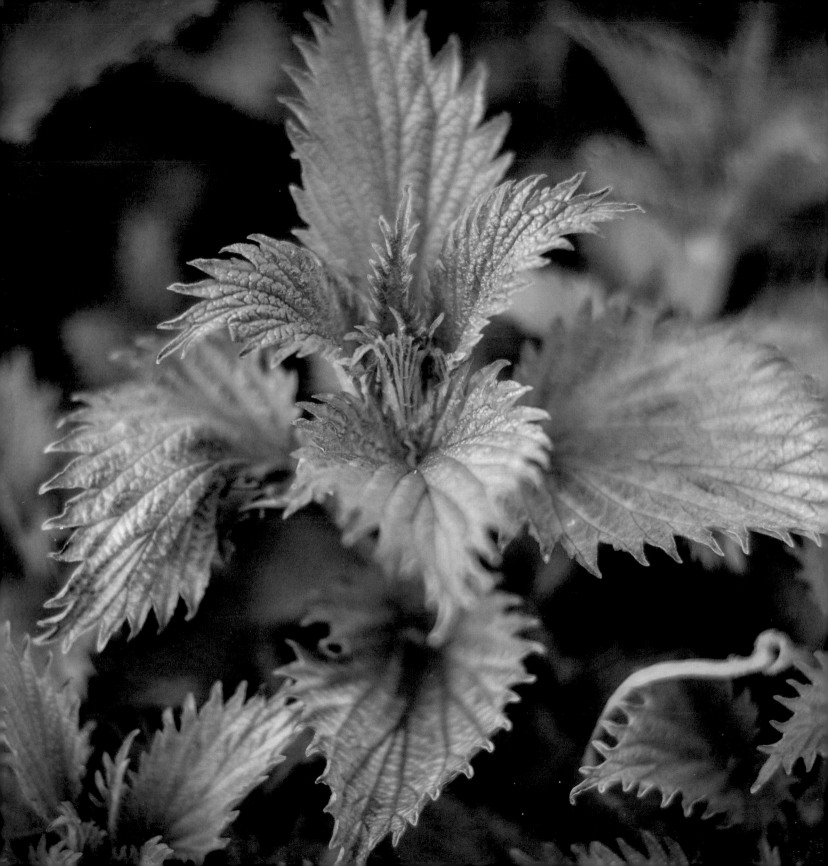

3 Nettle

Hello, friend! I'm so glad to see you again! It's a shame we can't shake hands or hug, but if you brush against my leaves and stems I could accidentally sting you. And I certainly don't want that.

You didn't think I would sting you on purpose, did you? Of course not! My stings were never meant for you. They help to keep me safe from animals who want to eat my leaves. If you do get stung, I'm very sorry for that.

Once we get to know each other better, stings will become rare. When you can recognize me from a distance you won't brush against me by mistake. Instead, you will learn how to harvest my leaves easily, without fear. Lean in close, you can see the sharp, fine hairs all over me that cause the sting. That's what you want to avoid.

While my scientific name, *Urtica dioica*, is rooted in the Latin word meaning "to burn," there is more to me than my sting. My leaves are packed with minerals and vitamins that your body needs. All it takes is drying, cooking, or pureeing to make them ready for eating.

I'm best for eating in early spring, and later in the year for tea. I'm only safe to eat before I flower, so don't wait! Cut me back midsummer and I'll give you another harvest later in the season. Use me for soups, teas, and other remedies, and I'll give you energy and nourish you more deeply than you ever dreamed! I do hope we can remain friends. Once you get to know me, you'll find so much love.

Latin Name:

Urtica dioica

Parts Used:
leaves, seeds, and roots

Energetics:
cool and dry

Nettle leaf is good for:

❋ Providing the body with abundant minerals, including iron, zinc, calcium, and magnesium

❋ Providing a gentle energy boost, without caffeine

❋ Soothing muscle aches and pains

❋ Nourishing the liver and kidneys

❋ Comforting the nervous system

❋ Strengthening the hair and scalp

❋ Easing seasonal allergies

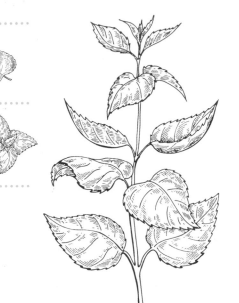

Field Identification

To identify nettle in the field, look for its key distinguishing characteristics. (Use the photograph on the right as a guide.)

Stem:
Nettle has a square stem and grows 2 to 4 feet high. Upon close inspection, you will find the stem is covered in sparse, prickly hairs.

Leaves:
Like its stem, nettle leaves are also covered in sparse, prickly hairs. Nettle leaves are oval at the base and pointed at the tip, with coarsely toothed edges. Each leaf emerges from a short stalk. They are arranged oppositely (in pairs) along the stem.

Flowers:
Because nettle is pollinated by the wind, not insects, the flowers are simple and nondescript. Green-to-yellow seedy, pollen-coated flowers ring the stem toward the top, arranged between the layers of leaves. While nettle leaves are not edible after flowering has begun, the seeds that ripen in mid to late summer are.

> **REMEMBER:** *Never consume nettle leaf after it has begun to flower.*

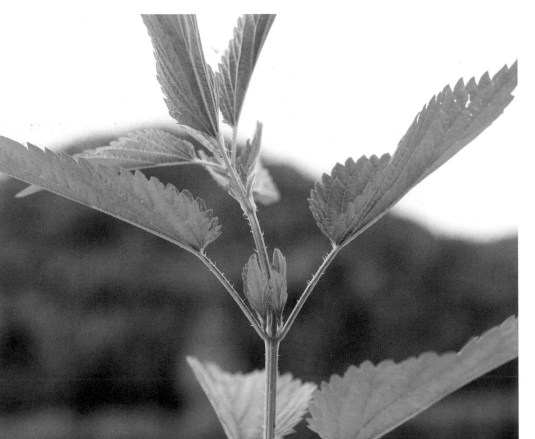

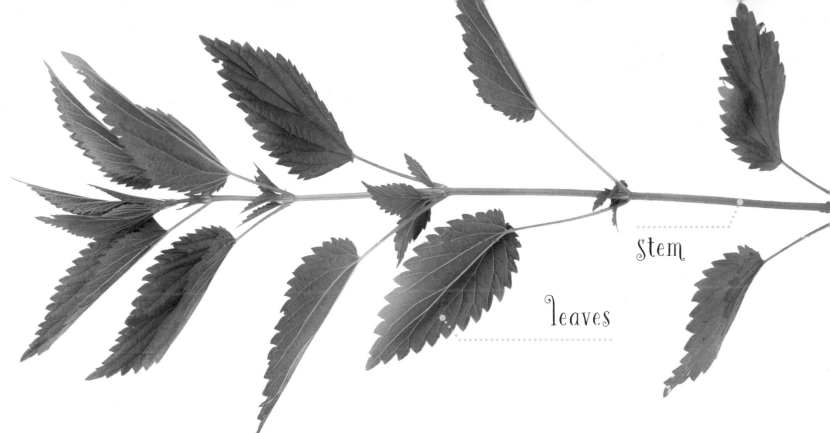

stem

leaves

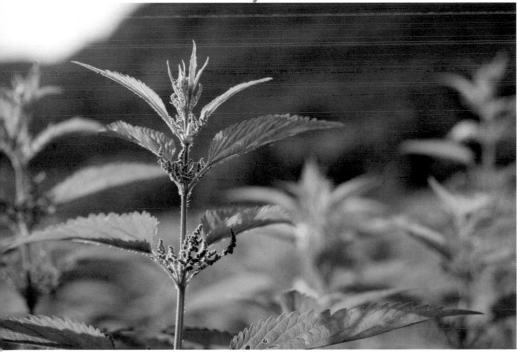

Growth habit:

Nettle loves to spread out, so you will rarely find a single nettle shoot growing alone. Spreading by both seed and root, nettle is frequently found in large clumps ranging from 1 to 10 feet across.

Habitat:

Nettle loves damp soil. It thrives along creek beds, in forests, in shady corners of empty lots, and in pastures.

Range:

Find nettle throughout all but the driest parts of North America, and in most areas worldwide.

Spring Nettle Soup

Creamy, delicious, and oh-so-nourishing, make this soup with the very first nettles of the season. When harvesting nettles for eating, choose only the four to six pairs of leaves found toward the plant's tender tip, as shown at right.

TIME: Less than 1 hour, not including foraging time	**YIELD:** 2 quarts

INGREDIENTS

- ❊ 1 medium clove of garlic
- ❊ 2 large potatoes
- ❊ 1 medium onion
- ❊ 6 to 8 ounces fresh nettle tips (If you don't have a kitchen scale, an average-sized cloth shopping bag loosely filled half to three-quarters full should suffice.)
- ❊ 2 tablespoons olive oil
- ❊ 1½ quarts chicken broth or vegetable stock
- ❊ Salt and pepper to taste
- ❊ Lemon wedges

Instructions

1. Peel and mince the garlic. Allow to rest for 5 to 10 minutes before heating, to activate the beneficial components of the garlic. (See page 149 for more information.)

2. Meanwhile, wash and coarsely chop the potatoes, and peel and chop the onion.

3. Prepare the nettle tips by placing them in a mixing bowl of cold water in the kitchen sink. Stir vigorously with a wooden spoon to remove most of the stinging hairs, making the leaves easier to handle.

4. Drain the nettles and finely chop, wearing kitchen gloves if desired. Remove any debris that snuck into your foraging bag, as well as any long or tough stems.

   SAFETY NOTE: Never puree very hot liquids, and always start slowly with the vent open on your blender lid. To do otherwise can cause the hot liquid to splash out of the blender and cause burns.

5. Sauté the onions in olive oil until translucent. Add the garlic and stir for a few seconds.

6. Add the potatoes, broth, salt, and pepper and simmer until the potatoes are tender.

7. Add the chopped nettle and stir. The nettle should wilt immediately, resembling cooked spinach. As soon as the nettle has wilted, remove from heat.

8. Allow the soup to cool for 15 to 30 minutes, and then carefully puree in batches using your blender. Puree until the soup is silky smooth, and then return to the pot to gently reheat. (I find that nettle clogs the openings in a submersible blender, even when I chop the leaves quite small. Therefore, I prefer using a regular blender for this recipe. Experiment and find the method that you prefer!)

Serve

Serve the nettle soup with a squeeze of fresh lemon.

Storage

Nettle soup will keep for 3 to 4 days in the refrigerator. Gently reheat before serving.

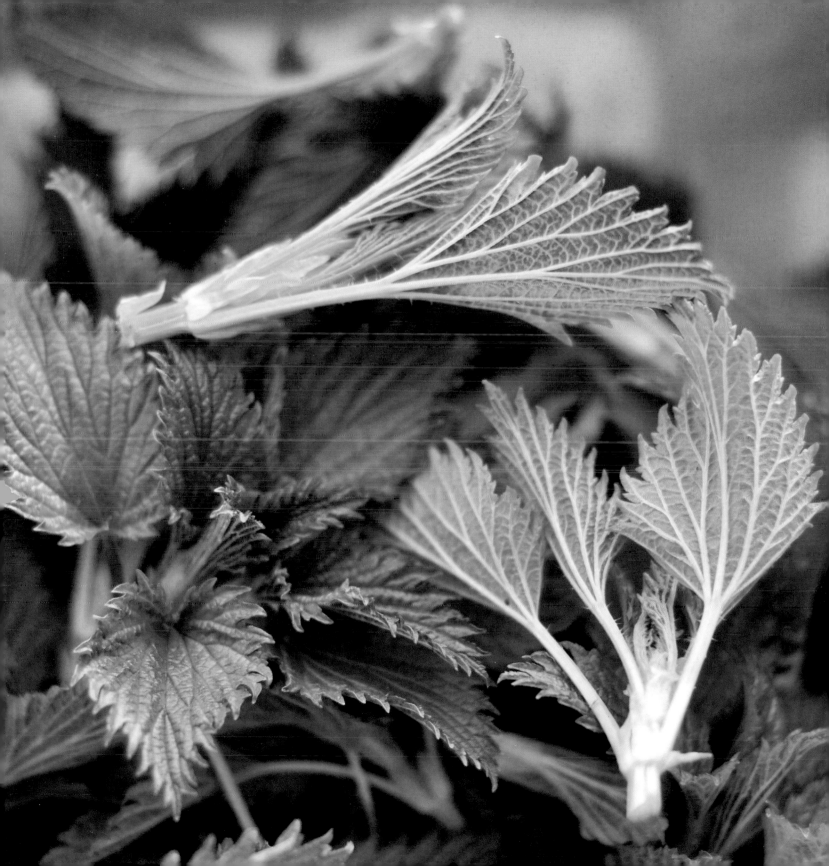

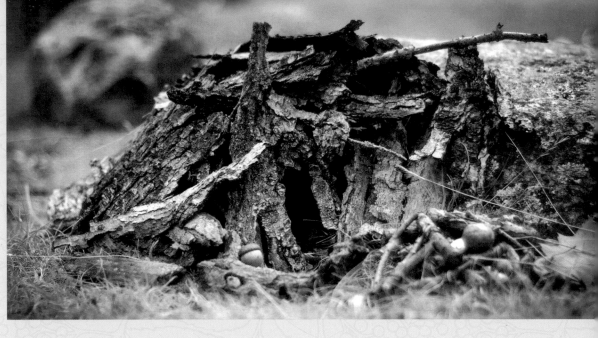

Only a vivid imagination and the building materials that nature provides are required! Look around the park, your yard, or garden shed to find building materials such as:

- ❋ Tree bark
- ❋ A hollow stump or log
- ❋ Twigs
- ❋ Leaves
- ❋ Moss
- ❋ Flat stones
- ❋ Clay or soil
- ❋ Seedpods
- ❋ Flower heads
- ❋ Clay pots
- ❋ And other inspiring bits of nature

Fairy Houses

Are there elves in the forest and fairies in your garden? I'd like to think so! Perhaps they help the spring flowers bloom and our garden veggies (and helpful weeds) grow. To encourage their garden magic, my family loves crafting fairy houses for them wherever we go. On the beach, in the backyard, and in the forest, perhaps the fairies discover our councesy handmade houses after we've gone back home ourselves . . .

Instructions

1. To build your fairy house, begin by gathering a variety of building materials.

2. Find a suitable, sheltered location to build your fairy house, based on the sort of fairy you want to attract. Flower fairies love to live at the edge of the flowerbed, birch fairies beneath a birch tree, garden gnomes beside the vegetable patch, and so on. Make sure your fairy house is out of the way of walking paths and lawnmowers.

3. Begin construction by following your inspiration. Create walls by pushing sticks into the soft earth, and then lining them with leaves or moss—or stack rocks to make a sturdy stone house. There is no right or wrong way to build a fairy house, as long as you follow your inspiration!

4. If desired, outfit your fairy house with improvised furniture and bedding crafted from twigs, leaves, and moss. We often leave little acorn caps full of fairy food inside, in case the wee folk are hungry for a snack when they get home!

Usha's Chai

INGREDIENTS

- 6 cups water
- 2 teaspoons cardamom seeds, or 2 tablespoons cardamom pods crushed with a mortar and pestle
- ⅓ teaspoon whole black peppercorns
- 7 whole cloves
- 2-inch knob of fresh ginger, thinly sliced
- ¼ cup shredded astragalus root (optional)
- 1 star anise pod
- 1 cinnamon stick, or 1 tablespoon cinnamon bark chips
- 1 very small pinch dried ground chili (optional)
- ¾ cup dried nettle leaf
- ¼ cup rooibos tea
- ¼ cup dried raspberry leaf (optional)
- Milk of your choice
- Coconut sugar (or other sweetener) to taste (1 to 3 teaspoons per cup, approximately)

If you've never tasted chai (spiced East Indian tea), you're in for a treat! Chai is flavorful, sweet, and easy to love. My friend Usha taught me how to make chai when I was a teenager, and I've been making a variation of her spiced Indian tea almost weekly ever since! Few things taste better to me than Usha's chai. (Except, perhaps, her cooking.) This version of the tea is caffeine-free.

ACTIVE TIME: Less than 20 minutes, not including foraging and drying time
TOTAL TIME: Less than 1 hour | **YIELD:** Approximately 8 servings

Instructions

1. In a medium cooking pot, combine the water with the cardamom, peppercorns, cloves, ginger, astragalus, anise, cinnamon, and chili. Place over high heat until it reaches a boil.

2. Reduce heat to low, cover, and simmer for 10 to 15 minutes.

3. Add the nettle leaf, raspberry leaf, and rooibos. Remove from heat and steep, covered, for 30 minutes.

4. Strain out and compost or discard your herbs, and then gently reheat your chai. To drink, combine 3 parts warm chai with 2 parts warm milk. Sweeten with a touch of coconut sugar or honey and enjoy!

Storage

Chai concentrate can be stored in the refrigerator for up to a week. Discard if it becomes sour.

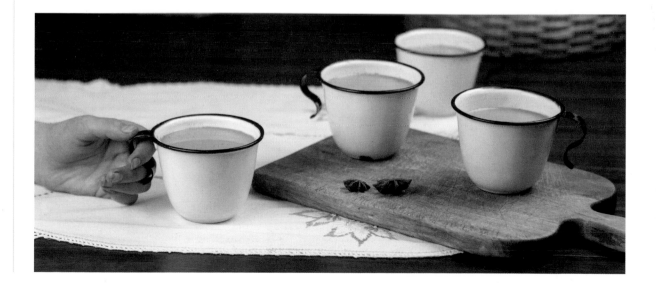

Mineral Magic Oxymel

Plants readily give up their minerals to vinegar, making it an ideal liquid for extracting plant nourishment. An oxymel (or vinegar-honey infusion) delivers not only the nutrition of the plants, but also of the goodness of raw vinegar and honey. Use the best-quality ingredients to create the best-quality remedy.

ACTIVE TIME: Less than 10 minutes, not including foraging and wilting or drying time
TOTAL TIME: 3 to 4 weeks | **YIELD:** 1¼ cup

INGREDIENTS

- 1½ cups wilted fresh nettle leaf, or 1 cup dried
- 1 cup raw apple cider vinegar
- ½ cup raw honey

Variation: Mineral Medley

Add other mineral-rich herbs to your infusion. Try substituting up to half of the nettle leaf with dandelion root, burdock root, raspberry leaf, chickweed, horsetail, oat straw, or kelp. For a different flavor, toss in some gingerroot or peppermint leaf. The possibilities are endless!

Instructions

1. Place the nettle leaf in clean, dry pint jar.

2. Pour the vinegar and honey over the nettle leaf and gently stir.

3. Push all the leaves beneath the surface of the liquid, and add additional vinegar or honey if needed. Be sure all the herbs are covered by 1 to 2 inches of liquid.

4. If the nettle leaves float, weigh them down with a clean, dry stone or smaller glass jar placed inside your pint jar.

5. Cover with a plastic lid or line the metal lid with parchment, waxed paper, or a plastic bag. Label the jar with the remedy name and date.

6. Store on a saucer in a dark place for 3 to 4 weeks.

7. During this time, remove the weight and shake or stir occasionally, pushing the leaves back under the surface if needed after shaking. Add additional honey or vinegar if needed to keep your plant material properly submerged.

8. After 3 to 4 weeks, strain your oxymel. Line a mesh colander with cheesecloth or clean muslin. Pour your remedy through this filter, and then twist the bundle tightly and squeeze with your hands to extract all the liquid that you can from the herbs.

9. Compost or discard the leaves, and transfer the oxymel to a clean, dry glass jar or bottle.

10. Lid and label.

To use

Adults can take 1 to 2 tablespoons daily or as desired; children can take 1 to 2 teaspoons daily. Stir into fizzy water or hot tea, drizzle over salads and cooked greens, or enjoy straight off the spoon.

Storage

Oxymels will keep for at least 1 year if stored in a cool, dark place.

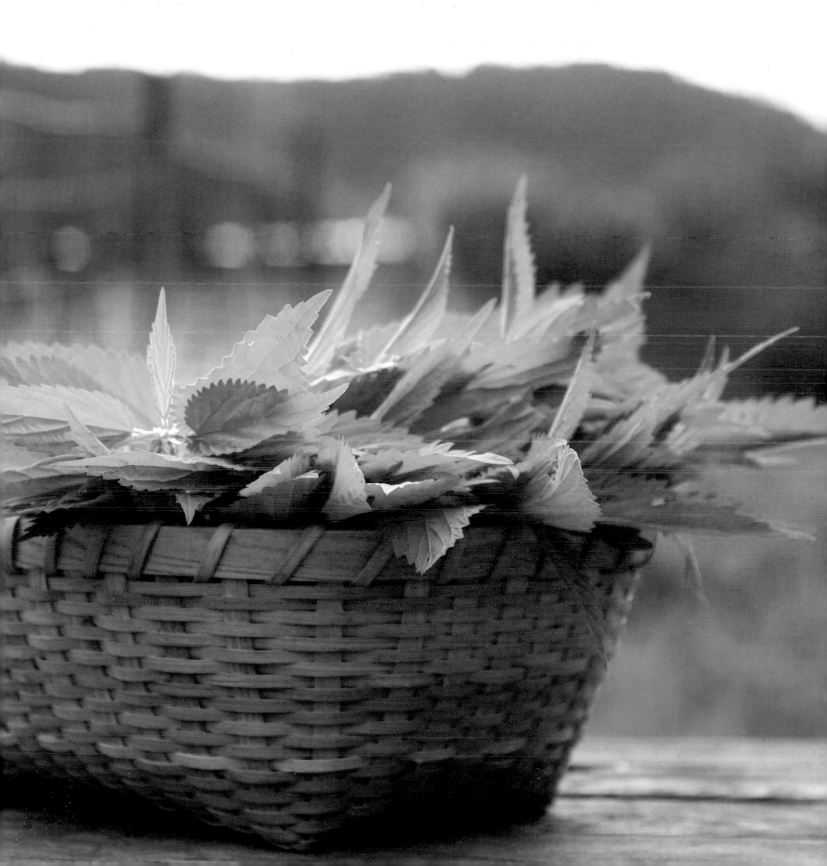

Popcorn Confetti

INGREDIENTS

- ½ cup dried nettle leaf
- ¼ cup nutritional yeast
- 1 tablespoon garlic powder
- 3 tablespoons dried dill weed
- 2 teaspoons fine sea salt
- ½ teaspoon finely ground pepper
- ½ cup popcorn
- 2 tablespoons coconut oil
- 3 tablespoons butter

My kids and I have been known to make a meal of popcorn and smoothies on more than one occasion. Somehow, adding Popcorn Confetti to the mix makes me feel like we're almost eating a healthy dinner. (Almost.) This popcorn topping is a delicious and nutritious addition to this favorite family snack.

TIME: Less than 15 minutes, not including foraging and drying time | **YIELD:** 1 cup

Instructions

1. Measure all the ingredients into a clean, dry mixing bowl.

2. Crush any large leaves between your fingers if necessary and stir well to combine.

3. Transfer to a spice jar with a shaker lid or a clean storage jar.

4. Lid and label.

To use

Make a bowl of popcorn, and then butter and sprinkle liberally with Popcorn Confetti. Devour and repeat! For best flavor, try popping ½ cup of popcorn in 2 tablespoons of coconut oil. Top with 3 tablespoons of butter and 2 to 4 tablespoons of Popcorn Confetti.

Storage

Stored in a cool dry place, Popcorn Confetti should last for 3 to 6 months.

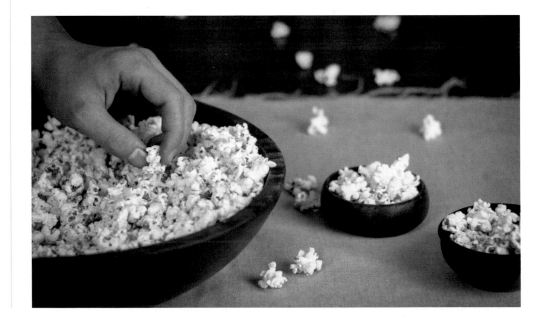

Herbal Hair Rinse

- ½ cup dried nettle leaf
- ¼ cup dried horsetail (optional)
- 2 tablespoons dried chamomile flowers
- 2 tablespoons dried lavender flowers
- 3½ cups raw apple cider vinegar
- 12 drops lavender essential oil (optional)

Bye-bye to tangles, and hello to healthy hair! Infused apple cider vinegar makes a wonderful after-shampoo rinse for smooth, shiny hair. It removes residues, tames dry, itchy scalps, and makes hair easier to comb.

ACTIVE TIME: Less than 10 minutes, not including foraging and drying time
TOTAL TIME: 6 to 8 weeks | **YIELD:** 3 cups

Instructions

1. Place the dried herbs and flowers in a quart-sized mason jar.

2. Cover with vinegar, making sure the herbs are completely submerged with no air pockets. Cover the herbs with a minimum of 2 inches of liquid. Stir well, pushing all the leaves beneath the surface of the liquid.

3. If your herbs float, weigh them down with a clean, dry stone or smaller glass jar placed inside your jar.

4. Cover with a plastic lid or line a metal lid with parchment, waxed paper, or a plastic bag.

5. Label the jar with the remedy name and date and store in a dark place for 3 to 4 weeks.

6. During this time, remove the weight and shake the jar occasionally, pushing the leaves back under the surface if needed after shaking. Add additional vinegar, if needed, to keep your plant material properly submerged.

7. After 3 to 4 weeks, strain your hair rinse. Line a mesh colander with cheesecloth or clean muslin. Pour your remedy through this filter, and then twist the bundle tightly and squeeze with your hands to extract all the liquid that you can from the herbs.

8. Compost or discard the leaves, and transfer the vinegar to a clean, dry glass jar or bottle.

9. Add lavender essential oil if desired.

10. Lid and label.

To use

Combine 1 part vinegar with 4 parts water in a plastic squeeze bottle. (An empty dish soap or shampoo bottle will work well.) Store your diluted vinegar mix in the shower for up to 2 weeks.

Shampoo as usual, rinse hair thoroughly, and apply a generous squirt of Herbal Hair Rinse to hair and scalp. Leave on hair and allow to air-dry. The vinegar scent disappears completely when hair is dry.

Storage

To prevent your hair rinse from spoiling, only dilute enough for approximately 2 weeks at a time. Wash and rinse your bottle well before each refill.

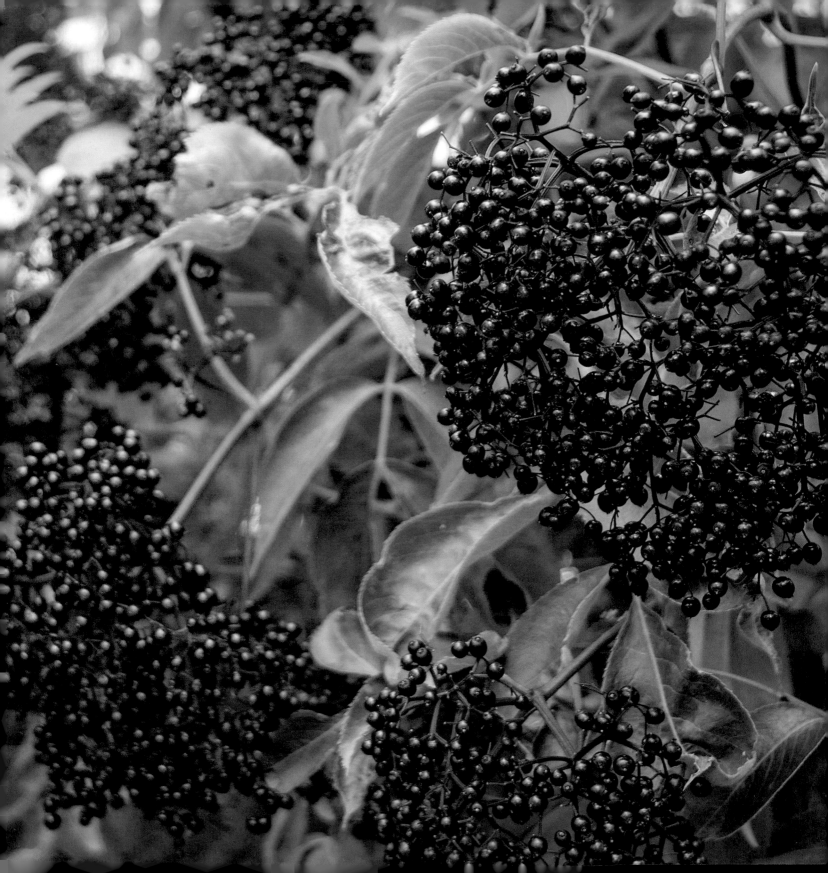

$\mathcal{Q}$ Elderberry

Hello, dear. How nice of you to visit! How about a cup of tea? (I'll add a bit of elderberry syrup, if you'd like.) And would you like some elderberry muffins for a snack?

I've known your family for so very long. Your great-great-grandmother used to harvest my flowers every summer for elderflower cordials and tea. She'd also gather my berries in August for elderberry syrup and wine. Oh my, yes. I've been around that long! Far longer, if you must know. Just how long, you ask? Now, now, dear. You know it isn't polite to ask the age of your elders.

I can tell you this—generations ago people believed that there was a spirit in each elder tree. An "elder woman" they called her. They'd even bring her gifts before they harvested, to make sure they stayed on her good side.

Today I don't see as many visitors as I used to. Will you come and visit me more often, dear? I'd like that. I can tell you my stories, and you can harvest my flowers and berries, just like your ancestors did. And no need to bring me gifts when you come. There's nothing I need aside from your company.

In case your great-great-grandmother didn't teach you about my uses, I'm happy to share them. In early summer, my flowers are a wonderful remedy for fevers, especially in children. In late summer, my berries ripen and they're useful for fighting colds, coughs, and flu—they're also delicious

Latin Name:

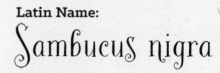

Sambucus nigra

Parts Used:
flowers and berries

Energetics:
cool and dry

Elder is a helpful herb for:
- ⚜ Treating fevers
- ⚜ Supporting the immune system
- ⚜ Fighting cold and flu
- ⚜ Treating coughs

baked into muffins, breads, and other treats. But don't eat my leaves or branches! They contain a poison that could make you feel sick. Eating my berries raw can also cause an upset stomach, so always cook, juice, or process before eating!

In some parts of the world elder is still a common remedy for cold and flu season. In regions of Europe, elderberry syrup is the most popular cold remedy you can find. But there's no need to *buy* elder syrup. You can make your own from scratch with my fresh, frozen, or dried berries.

Do come visit again soon, my dear. It's been so nice to see you.

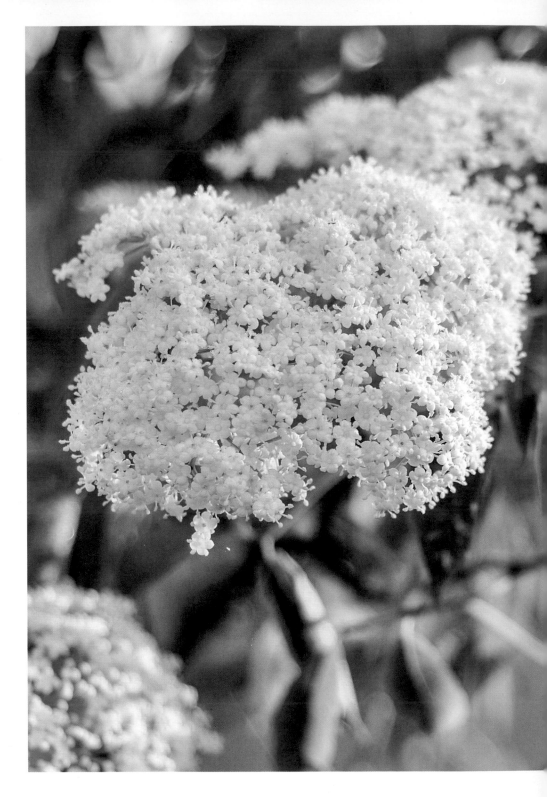

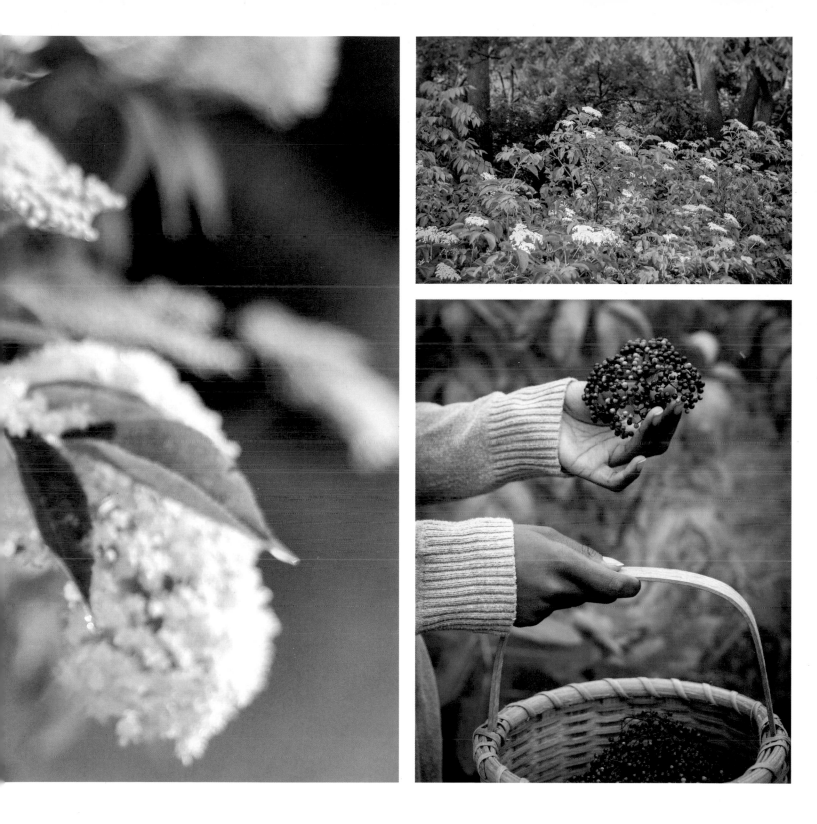

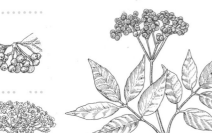

Field Identification

To identify elderberry in the field, look for its key distinguishing characteristics. (Use the photographs below and at right as a guide.)

Stem:
Elderberry stems are covered in a smooth, brown bark, marked with many raised bumps (called lenticels). Branching is opposite, with leaves and branches emerging in pairs opposite one another along the stem. Elder branches are brittle and hollow and contain a soft, white pith.

Leaves:
Elderberry leaves are compound, bearing five to nine leaflets each. Leaves are "pinnate," which means the leaflets are arranged along its length in pairs. A single terminal leaflet completes the tip. Leaf edges are serrated.

Flowers:
Creamy white flowers are produced in umbrella-shaped clusters, called umbels. Umbels range in size from 4 to 8 inches. Each tiny flower has five rounded petals and five protruding stamens (male flower parts).

leaves

stem

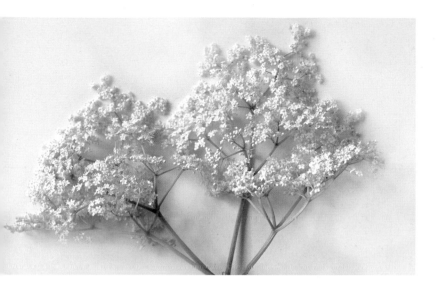

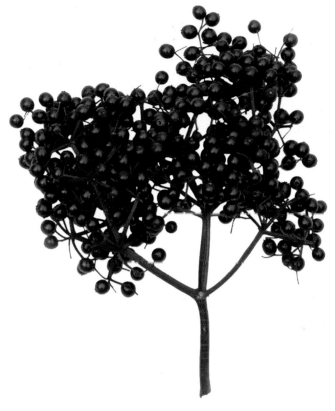

> **NOTE:** *Both fresh and dried elderberry leaves and stems are poisonous if consumed. (The leaves, however, are used as a topical remedy.) Berries can cause upset stomach or vomiting when eaten raw, so always cook or infuse your elderberries into liquid before consuming.*

Berries:

Umbel-shaped clusters of berries are concentrated across the top of the bush. The fruit clusters commonly droop downward from the weight of the berries. When ripe, the berries are deep purple to black.

Growth habit:

Elderberry is a woody shrub growing 8 to 9 feet tall. Many branches often emerge from the same root, producing a dense cluster of bushes. The bark of new young shoots is green and tender, while established plants have pronounced lenticels (pores) peppered across the otherwise smooth, brown bark.

Habitat:

Elderberries like moist soil and plenty of sunshine. You'll find them along wetland edges and creek banks, roadsides, and moist fields.

Range:

Elderberry is found throughout most of North America and Europe.

Lookalikes:

While elderberry has no convincing lookalikes, it shares qualities with other species in flower type, leaf shape, or berry color.

Deadly water hemlock, for example, also bears creamy white flowers in an umbrella-like shape and has compound, toothed leaves.

Water hemlock, however, is an herbaceous, or non-woody, plant that lacks the brown bark seen on elderberry bushes. Pokeweed bears poisonous berries a similar color to elderberry, but it lacks the compound leaves and umbrella-shaped berry clusters of elder.

Elderberry reminds us to positively identify our plants before harvest. Always check bark, leaves, *and* flowers or berries before determining if you have found the plant you seek.

Natural Dyes for Silk or Wool

What do red cabbage, dandelion leaves, elderberries, and dried black beans have in common? No, they're not the ingredients for a strange new casserole, though all *can* be used in food recipes. Each one is also a colorful dye for silk and wool.

SUPPLIES

- ❧ Up to 6 undyed play silks or other 100-percent silk or wool fabric, or 3 small skeins of 100-percent wool or silk yarn
- ❧ 14 cups water, divided
- ❧ ½ cup table salt *or* ½ teaspoon alum powder (see "Prepare your fabric")
- ❧ 2 to 4 cups fresh or dried elderberries, black walnut husks, or dry black beans *or* 5 to 6 cups chopped leaves and/or flowers of your choice (most leaves and flowers yield yellow dye)

Instructions

The colors produced with natural dyes are subtle and earthy. Unlike synthetic dyes, you never know exactly what color will emerge from the dye pot until your project is done. Experiment with foraged dyes, such as elderberry, dandelion, goldenrod, and tansy. Or dream up dyes from the kitchen, such as red cabbage, turmeric, dried black beans, or blueberries.

> **NOTE:** Though it is possible to use natural dyes to color 100-percent cotton fabrics in very subtle pastel shades, both silk and wool take color more enthusiastically and yield more satisfying results.

Prepare your fabric.

1. For natural dyes to properly adhere to fibers, the fabric must first be soaked in a solution that prepares it to absorb the dye. This solution is called a mordant. An alum mordant will result in slightly deeper hues, but for more pastel shades, simple table salt works as well. The choice is yours.

2. Place 8 cups of water in a nonreactive pan and set over high heat. Bring to a simmer and add the table salt *or* alum.

3. Stir to dissolve the mordant and remove the pot from the heat.

4. Place your fabric or yarn in the pot and gently submerge. Do not stir vigorously if you are working with wool, as it may become felted through the agitation!

5. Cover and allow to soak for 1½ hours. Make your dye bath using the following instructions while your fabric soaks.

6. Remove the fabric or yarn with a spoon, and then rinse gently but thoroughly in tap water of roughly the same temperature as your mordant bath.

Make your dye bath.

1. Combine your plant material with 6 cups of water in a large stainless steel pot.

2. Cover and gently warm over low heat for 1 hour, stirring occasionally. It should barely reach a simmer.

3. Remove the pot from the heat, remove the cover, and allow the dye bath to cool for 30 minutes.

4. Carefully pour the liquid through a cheesecloth-lined strainer, reserving the liquid. Discard the solids.

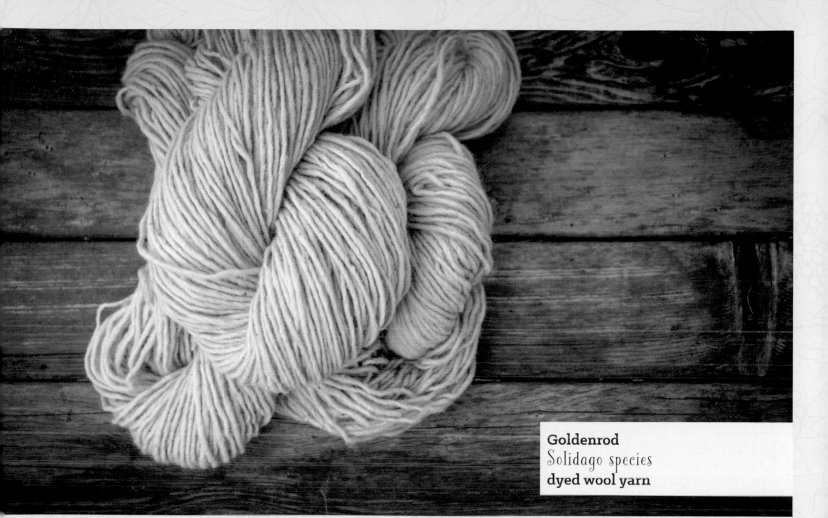

Goldenrod
Solidago species
dyed wool yarn

Dye your fabric!

1. Heat your dye solution until very hot but not yet simmering, and then remove from the heat.

2. Add your prepared fabric and submerge it in the dye with a stainless steel or plastic spoon.

3. Cover and allow to steep between 1½ hours and overnight, gently stirring on occasion. (The longer you steep, the more vibrant your colors will be. Be patient!)

4. Gently rewarm the dye bath as needed if it becomes cold. However, never boil your fabric, as it could damage the fibers.

5. When you are pleased with the color of your silk or wool, remove it from the dye bath and rinse well. Hang to dry.

Elderberry Syrup

Elderberry syrup is your secret cold-fighting weapon! Best of all? It's lip-smacking delicious.

INGREDIENTS

- ¾ cup (approximately 3 ounces) dried elderberries
- 5 cups water
- 2 tablespoons dried rose hips
- 1 cinnamon stick
- 2 teaspoons whole clove
- 1-inch piece of fresh ginger root, sliced
- 1¼ cups raw honey

ACTIVE TIME: 1½ hours, not including foraging and drying time
TOTAL TIME: approximately 2½ hours | **YIELD:** 4½ cups

Instructions

1. Combine all ingredients except honey in a large, stainless steel cooking pot.

2. Simmer over medium heat until the volume of water is reduced by approximately 50 percent, approximately 20 to 30 minutes. The color will be deep and rich.

3. Remove from heat and cool until just warm to the touch.

4. Pour mixture through a fine mesh strainer. Press or squeeze berries to extract as much juice as possible. Compost or discard solids.

5. Add additional water if needed to bring your volume back up to 2½ cups.

6. Add honey, and stir well to combine.

7. Bottle, label, and store in the refrigerator.

To use

Take 1 teaspoon for children, 1 tablespoon for adults daily throughout cold and flu season. If you feel a cold coming on, increase dosage to 1 to 2 teaspoons every 4 hours for up to 4 days for children, and 1 to 2 tablespoons every 4 hours for adults.

Storage

Stored in the refrigerator, elderberry syrup should last for 6 months.

TIP: *Always used dried elderberries for this recipe, as fresh ones will yield weaker, watery syrup.*

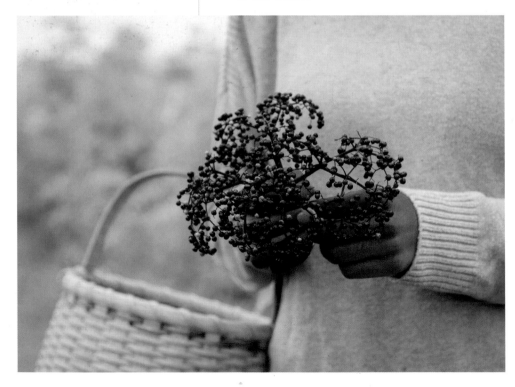

Elderberry Gummies

Don't get these herbal treats confused with the gummies you might buy at the candy store! Unlike their sweet-and-sour candy store cousins, elderberry gummies are far more mild—and nourishing. Delicious and easy to eat, they're a delightful way to enjoy your daily dose of elderberries.

ACTIVE TIME: Less than 20 minutes, not including foraging and drying
TOTAL TIME: 2 hours | **YIELD:** One 8×8 pan of gummies

INGREDIENTS

- ½ cup (approximately 2 ounces) dried elderberries
- 3 cups water
- 1 tablespoon fresh lemon juice, or ¼ cup orange juice concentrate
- ¼ cup grass-fed gelatin powder
- ¼ cup raw honey

TIP: Always use dried elderberries for this recipe, as fresh ones will yield weaker, watery gummies.

Instructions

1. Combine the water and dried berries in a medium pot.

2. Simmer over medium heat until the volume of water is reduced by 25 to 50 percent. The color will be deep and rich.

3. Remove from heat and cool slightly.

4. Add the lemon juice, stir, and pour the mixture through a fine-mesh strainer. Press or squeeze the berries to extract as much juice as possible. Compost or discard the solids.

5. Add additional water, if needed, to bring your volume back up to 1½ cups.

6. Whisk the gelatin into the still-warm liquid by hand, and then stir in the honey. (Do not use an electric mixer or blender, which will compromise the texture of the finished gummies.)

7. Pour into an 8×8 baking dish or gummy molds.

8. Transfer carefully to the refrigerator and chill until fully set.

9. Cut and eat!

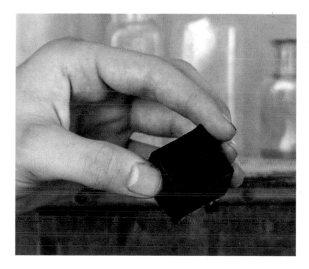

To use

Enjoy these gummies as a snack or dessert. Eat a few 1-inch cubes per day, as desired. Because these gummies contain honey, they are not suitable for children under one year of age.

Storage

Gummies are so delicious that they never last long! Store in the refrigerator for up to 4 days.

Strawberry-Elderflower Soda Syrup

Soda from the grocery store has nothing on this! Make your own sweet fizzy drinks by crafting a fruity-floral syrup and adding it to fizzy water. You might never reach for a can of soda again. But don't wait! Neither elderflower nor strawberry season lasts long.

ACTIVE TIME: Less than 30 minutes, not including foraging time.
TOTAL TIME: 24 hours | **YIELD:** 2 cups

INGREDIENTS

- ✻ 10 medium-sized (approximately 6 inches across) fresh elderflower umbels (approximately 2½ cups of flowers)
- ✻ ½ organic lemon (with the peel), thinly sliced
- ✻ 1 teaspoon fresh, grated gingerroot
- ✻ 2¼ cups water, divided
- ✻ 2 cups (approximately 8 ounces) fresh or frozen strawberries, sliced
- ✻ ⅓ to ½ cup raw honey or sugar

Instructions

1. Harvest elderflowers on the same day you will make your syrup. Pick blooms after the morning dew has dried, but before the heat of the day. Choose clusters where most buds are open; avoid clusters with flowers tinged with brown and already past their prime. These spent flowers will taint the flavor of your finished syrup.

2. To harvest, snap or cut off the whole umbels (clusters) of flowers and place them gently into your harvest basket. Back home, pick over the flowers for insects, debris, and any browned blossoms. Discard debris. Do not wash or rinse the flowers, as you will rinse away some of the fragrant nectar!

3. Remove any large stems, and then fill a quart-sized mason jar with the elderflowers, ginger, and lemon.

4. Boil 1½ cups of water and pour over the elderflowers.

5. Stir and loosely cover. Allow to steep on the counter overnight.

6. The next morning pour the syrup through a fine-mesh strainer. Press to extract as much syrup from the flowers as possible. Compost or discard the solids.

7. Meanwhile, place the sliced strawberries in a small saucepan. Combine with ¾ cup of water and bring to a simmer over medium-low heat.

8. Simmer for 5 minutes and mash berries with the back of a spoon.

9. Remove from heat and steep covered for 30 minutes.

10. Pour the strawberry-infused water through a fine-mesh strainer. Press to extract as much liquid as you can and reserve the berry pulp for another use, or compost or discard.

11. Stir the honey or sugar into the strawberry infusion until dissolved, and then combine with the elderflower infusion.

To use

Combine 1 part syrup with 2 parts carbonated water. Adjust proportions as desired and serve over ice.

Storage

Strawberry-Elderflower Soda Syrup will keep for up to 1 week in the refrigerator or 1 year in the freezer.

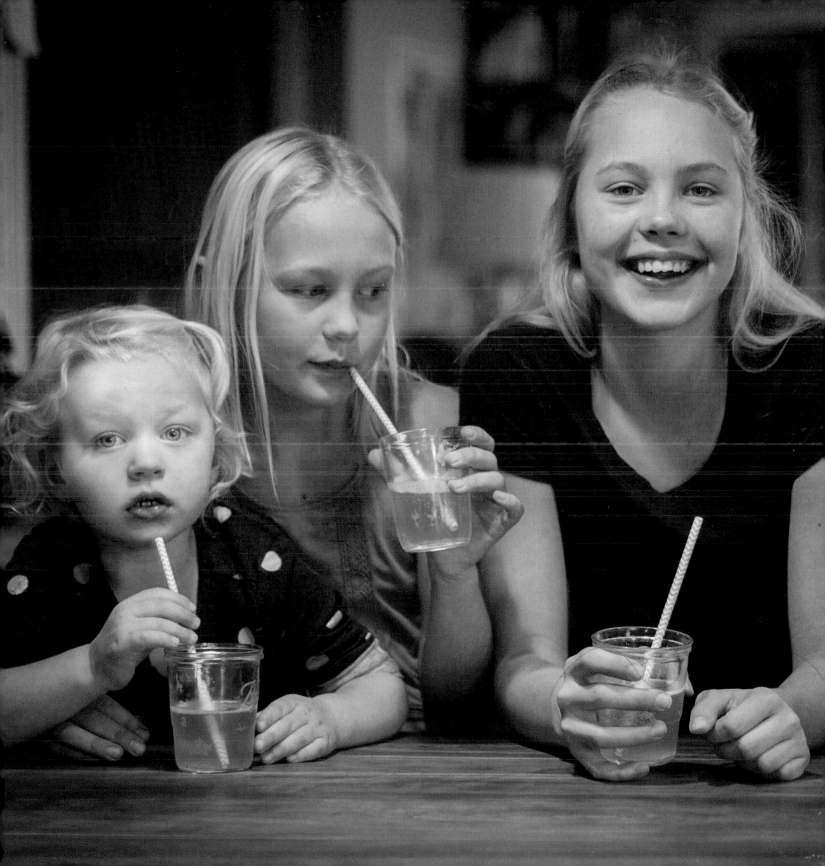

Elderflower Honey

Stir this flavorful honey into winter teas or cups of warm milk, drizzle on buttered toast, or enjoy right off the spoon. Perfect for cold season, sore throats, fevers, or anytime you crave a delicious treat that tastes of summer.

ACTIVE TIME: Less than 10 minutes, not including foraging time
TOTAL TIME: 3 weeks | **YIELD:** 1 scant pint

INGREDIENTS

- 6 to 10 umbels of ripe elderflowers
- 1 pint raw honey

Instructions

1. Harvest elderflowers on the same day you will make your syrup. Pick blooms after the morning dew has dried, but before the heat of the day. Choose clusters where most buds are open and avoid clusters with flowers tinged with brown and already past their prime. These spent flowers will taint the flavor of your finished syrup.

2. To harvest, snap or cut off the whole umbels (clusters) of flowers and place them gently into your harvest basket.

3. Back home, pick over the flowers for insects, debris, and any browned blossoms. Do not wash or rinse flowers.

4. Using scissors or your fingers, remove the blossoms from the stems, cutting or pulling away as much stem as possible. (A few stray bits of stem are fine, but remove what you can, including all large stems.)

5. Place the flowers in a clean, dry pint jar, filling nearly full without packing.

6. Pour raw honey over the blooms and use a table knife to remove air bubbles by gently stirring.

7. Lid, label, and place the jar in a dark cupboard for 2 to 3 weeks. Stir daily or when you think of it.

8. After the infusing period is up, pour the honey through a colander lined with several layers of cheesecloth.

9. Squeeze to extract as much honey as possible and compost or discard the spent blooms. Lid and label your elderflower honey with the remedy type and date.

To use

Use as you would plain honey—on toast, in tea, or in warm porridge. Or enjoy directly off the spoon for sore throats, coughs, and fevers. Because this remedy contains honey, it is not suitable for children under 1 year of age.

Storage

Stored in a cool, dry place, Elderflower Honey will keep for at least 1 year.

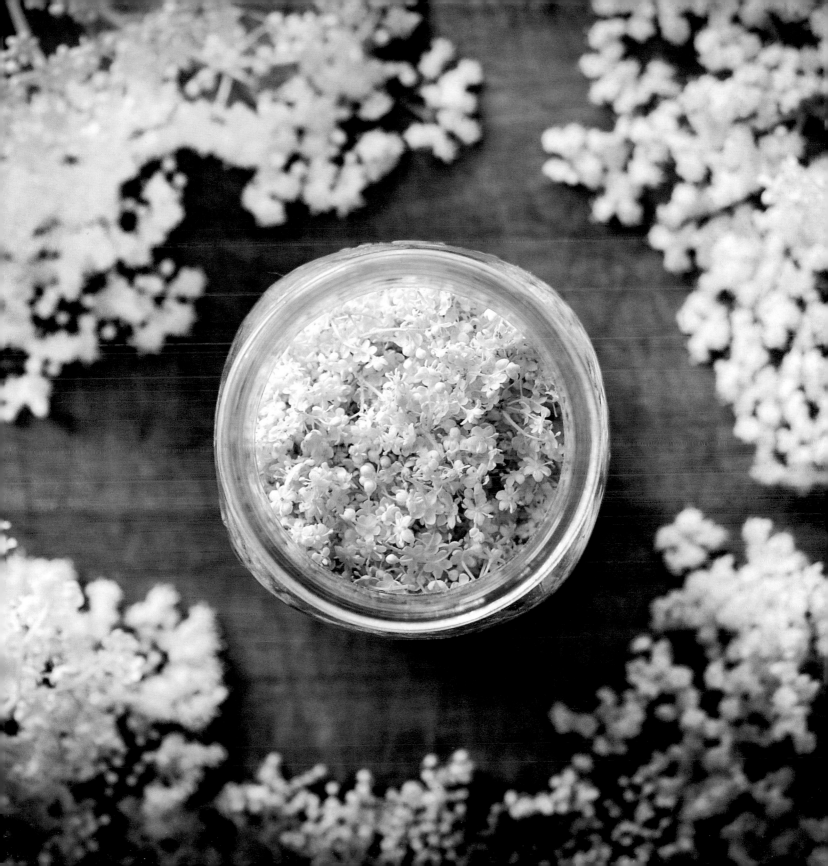

Elderberry Switchel

INGREDIENTS

- ⅓ cup raw apple cider vinegar
- ½ cup fresh or frozen elderberries, or ¼ cup dried
- ⅓ cup maple syrup or raw honey
- 1½ tablespoons fresh, grated gingerroot
- Approximately 2 quarts fresh water

A sweet and tangy treat, switchel might be the original soft drink. Made with apple cider vinegar, fresh ginger, and honey, it's the most delicious way to stay hydrated on a hot summer day. Switchel recipes date back at least to the early days of the US colonies, and have been enjoyed in North America for hundreds of years. (Laura Ingalls Wilder and Pa drink switchel while haying in the book *The Long Winter*.) My version includes elderberries for an immune-boosting punch. Add a pinch of unrefined sea salt and baking soda, and it makes a wonderful alternative to sports drinks.

ACTIVE TIME: Less than 20 minutes, not including foraging or drying time
TOTAL TIME: 12 hours | **YIELD:** 2 quarts

Instructions

1. Combine the elderberries, ginger, honey or maple syrup, and vinegar in a half-gallon mason jar, or divide evenly between two quart-sized jars.

2. Muddle the berries with the back of a wooden spoon, pressing gently to release some juices.

3. Fill with water to the shoulders and stir to combine.

4. Cover and refrigerate overnight. (You can rush it, but the flavor won't be as nice.)

5. Strain, taste for sweetness and adjust if desired, and serve.

Storage

Switchel will keep for 4 days in the refrigerator.

Variation

Experiment with adding other seasonal herbs and berries as well, such as rinsed staghorn sumac berries, fresh wild raspberries, or foraged mint. (If you are using sumac berries, strain them through a flour sack towel to remove the hairs.)

Apple cider vinegar may not be suitable for some individuals with acid reflux, heartburn, or indigestion.

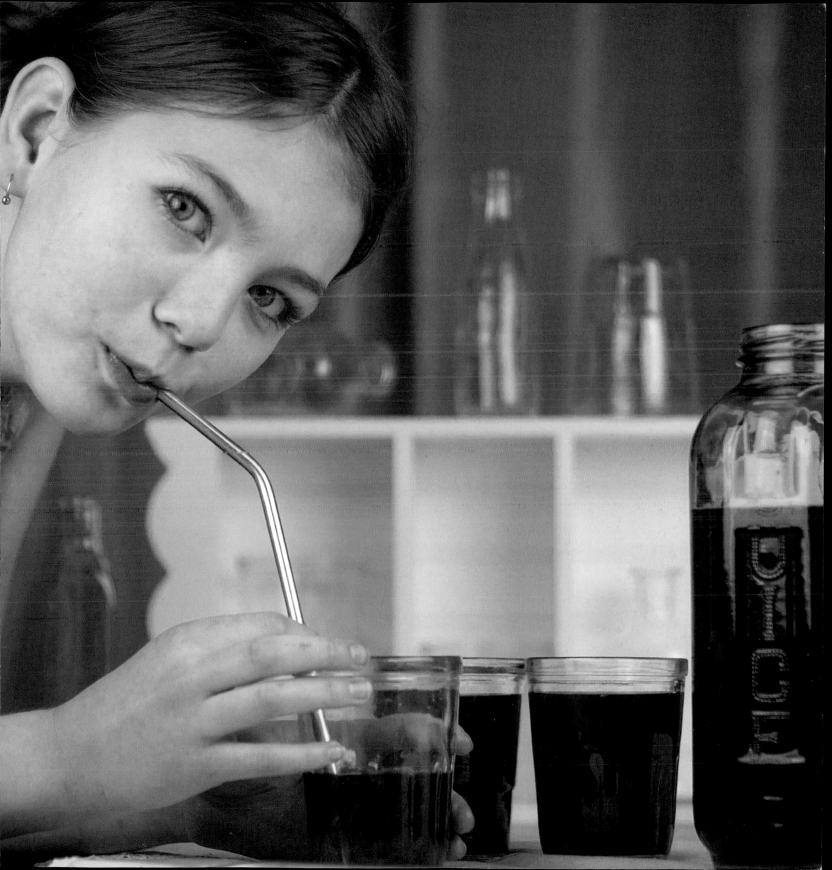

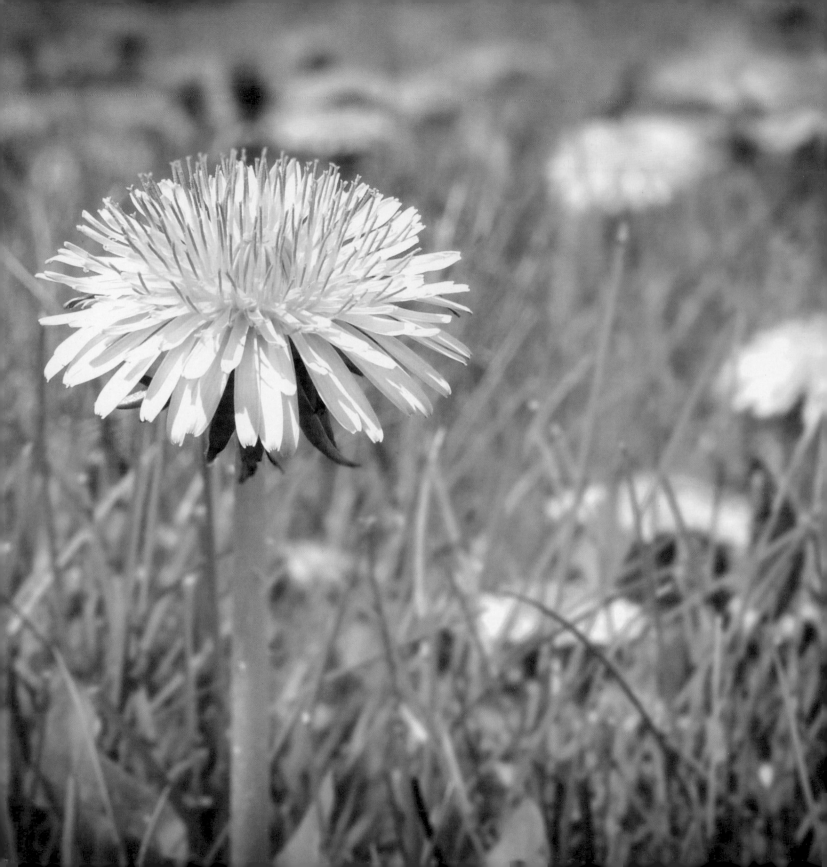

5 Dandelion

Hey, friend! How've you been? We've known each other for almost forever, haven't we? I've always felt our friendship was pretty special, since I'm the one you whisper your wishes to. (I hope they've all come true!)

I remember when you were just a little one, constantly popping things in your mouth that didn't belong. Now and then you may have even tasted my flowers, but I don't think you knew what to make of them! My flowers *are* bitter, I know. Everything about me is bitter—except for my sunny disposition. My flowers, leaves, and roots are all famous for their intensely bitter flavor. But they are good medicine, I assure you! And good food too, once you learn how to prepare them.

Bitter tastes like mine are *so good* for you. Even if you don't think that bitter is tasty, it's the flavor that tells your digestive system to wake up and get to work. Bitter tastes like mine turn on your saliva flow and fire up the stomach acid and the juices throughout your digestive tract. That means you get more nutrients from the food you eat and have fewer stomachaches and bathroom troubles.

And when you have less tummy trouble and absorb more nutrients, that means you have more energy to think, work, and play. Once you get to know me for more than my flowers, I think you'll discover that despite (or because of!) my bitter taste, there's much more of me to love.

Latin Name:

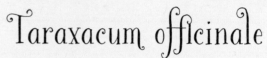
Taraxacum officinale

Parts Used:
roots, leaves, and flowers

Energetics:
cool and dry

Dandelion is a helpful herb for:
- Promoting healthy digestion
- Supplying high amounts of vitamins A, C, and K, iron, and calcium
- Supporting healthy liver function
- Gently acting as a diuretic
- Easing constipation
- Supplying antioxidants

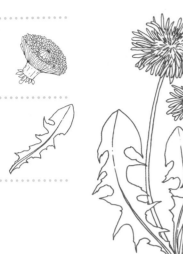

Field Identification

To identify dandelion in the field, look for its key distinguishing characteristics. (Use the photograph on the right as a guide.)

Stem:
Dandelion stems are hollow and exude a milky, white sap when broken.

Leaves:
The name "dandelion" is derived from the French phrase *dent de lion* or "tooth of the lion" for its deeply lobed, jagged-edged leaves. A close look at the leaves will show you why. Dandelion leaves are smooth and dark green, narrow at the base, and wider toward the tip. The surface of the leaf is completely free of hair or fuzz, distinguishing it from lookalike plants.

Flowers:
Dandelion flowers are easily recognizable. They are a composite-type flower, with each flower head made up of thousands of tiny flowers called ray florets. Each tiny ray floret forms a seed after the flower has bloomed and faded. Unlike lookalike species, each hollow dandelion stem bears only a single flower.

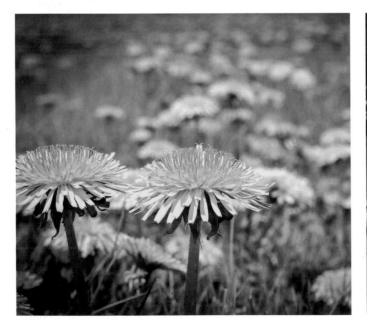

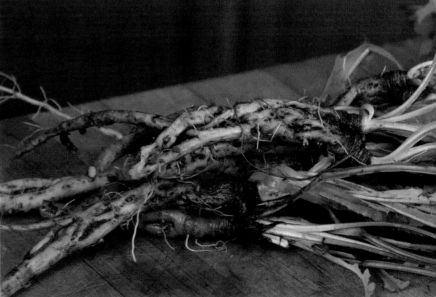

Avoid dandelion in cases of severe diarrhea, kidney stones, stomach inflammation or ulcers, gallbladder disease, gallstones, acid reflux, and bile-duct obstruction. During pregnancy, consume dandelion only in food in small quantities, and avoid extractions.

Root:

Dandelion grows from a sturdy, multi-branched taproot. The outside is tan, while the inside of the root is white.

Growth habit:

Dandelions grow from a basal rosette (or rose-shaped cluster of leaves), with a ring of leaves encircling one or more lower stems.

Habitat:

Dandelions are adaptable plants that grow nearly anywhere! You will find them in open fields, lawns, city lots, and roadsides. Dandelions can thrive in a wide variety of habitats, soil types, and climates.

Range:

Dandelions are native to Europe and Asia and are now found throughout most regions of North America.

Lookalikes:

Dandelion has several lookalikes, including cat's-ear, hawkweed, and shepherd's purse. None of these

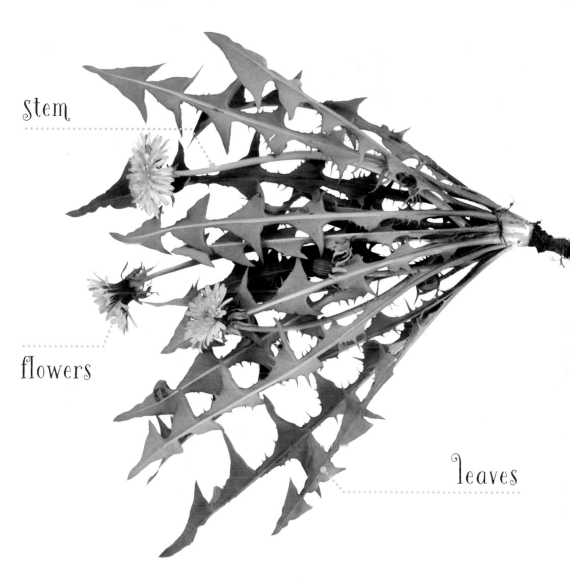

lookalikes are dangerous, but it's important to know you have the right plant any time you go out to forage.

It is easy to distinguish dandelion from other species by double-checking these key dandelion characteristics:

Leaves are smooth and hairless. Look closely for any sign of hairs or a fuzzy bloom on either side of the leaf. If hairs are present you have a different species.

Stems are hairless, hollow, and exude a milky sap when broken; other species lack these characteristics.

There is one bud or flower per stem; if more than one flower or bud is present, you have a lookalike, not a dandelion.

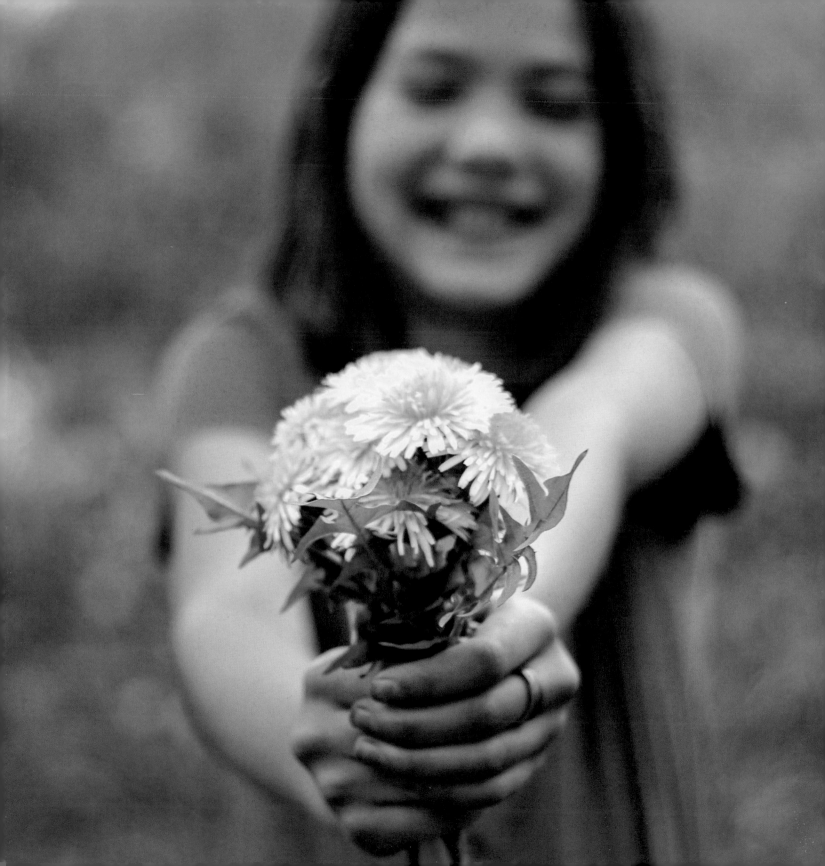

Dandelion Fritters

- 1 cup freshly picked dandelion flowers
- ¾ cup all-purpose flour
- ⅛ teaspoon salt
- ½ cup corn flour or finely ground cornmeal
- 1 teaspoon cinnamon
- 1 egg
- 2 tablespoons milk
- 1 tablespoon maple syrup
- Coconut oil or ghee for frying

Dandelion fritters are a tasty summertime treat. Made with whole dandelion flowers dipped in a pancake batter, they seem like something the garden fairies might enjoy! Keep in mind that the green base of the dandelion flower is the most bitter part. If you'd like a milder treat, remove the petals from your dandelions and add them into your batter, rather than dipping the whole flower heads. Then fry up your petal-specked fritters like pancakes.

TIME: Less than 20 minutes, not including foraging time | **YIELD:** 4 servings

Instructions

1. Harvest dandelion flowers after the morning dew has dried. Pick over your harvest and remove any garden debris.

2. Remove the green leaves (called sepals) growing on the undersides of the flowers by cutting or pulling off the stem-end of the blossoms. (This makes for tastier fritters, but it is not necessary.) If you cut off too much of the flower the head will fall apart, so experiment until you find a method that works best for you.

3. Set the trimmed blossoms aside.

4. In a medium-sized mixing bowl, combine the flour, salt, corn flour or cornmeal, and cinnamon. Whisk to combine.

5. In a separate bowl beat the egg with the milk and maple syrup.

6. Pour the wet ingredients into the dry ingredients and stir until just combined.

7. Heat the cooking oil in a cast iron or nonstick skillet over medium-high heat.

8. Grasp a flower by the base and dip into batter to coat. Carefully place petal-side down in the frying pan. Repeat until the pan is full but not crowded. Cook until golden brown, and then flip, and cook the second side.

9. Repeat with the remaining flowers and serve immediately with honey or maple syrup.

Allergy-Friendly Variations

Dandelion fritters can easily be made without common allergens! Use any or all of the substitutions below to meet your family's dietary needs.

- **Gluten-free:** Substitute a gluten-free flour blend of your choice for the flour.

- **Dairy-free:** Substitute coconut or almond milk for the cow milk in the original recipe.

- **Egg-free:** Omit the egg, instead combining 1 tablespoon ground flax or chia seed with 2½ tablespoons water. Allow to sit for 10 minutes, and then proceed with the recipe.

- **Corn-free:** Replace cornmeal with almond flour.

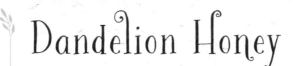

Dandelion Honey

Flower-infused honey is the bee's knees! This dandelion-infused syrup tastes just like a summer day. A fun, simple project for even the smallest of hands.

ACTIVE TIME: Less than 20 minutes, not including foraging and wilting time
TOTAL TIME: 4 weeks | **YIELD:** 1 cup

INGREDIENTS

- ❁ 2 cups freshly harvested dandelion flowers
- ❁ 1¼ cups honey, or enough to cover flowers

Instructions

1. Harvest fresh, vibrant dandelion heads after the morning dew has dried. Pick over your harvest and remove any garden debris.

2. Using your fingers, pull the petals from the green flower base. Compost or discard the green portion and set the petals aside. Your harvest should yield approximately 1 cup of petals. Don't fret if you end up with more or less. This recipe adapts to any quantity.

3. When all of your flowers have been processed, set them aside to wilt for 12 to 24 hours.

4. After wilting, transfer your dandelion petals to a half-pint jar. The flower petals should fill the jar approximately half to two-thirds full. If you harvested a different quantity of petals, simply choose a smaller or larger jar, as needed.

5. Pour raw honey over the petals, filling the jar to the shoulders. Lid and label.

6. Set on a counter out of direct sun for 4 to 6 weeks, and slowly turn the jar over to mix every few days.

7. Strain the honey through a fine-mesh strainer, squeezing as much liquid goodness as you can out of the petals. Compost or discard the solids.

To use

Stir into warm tea, drizzle on pancakes, or sneak a little right off the spoon!

Storage

Stored in a cool, dry place, Dandelion Honey will keep for at least 1 year.

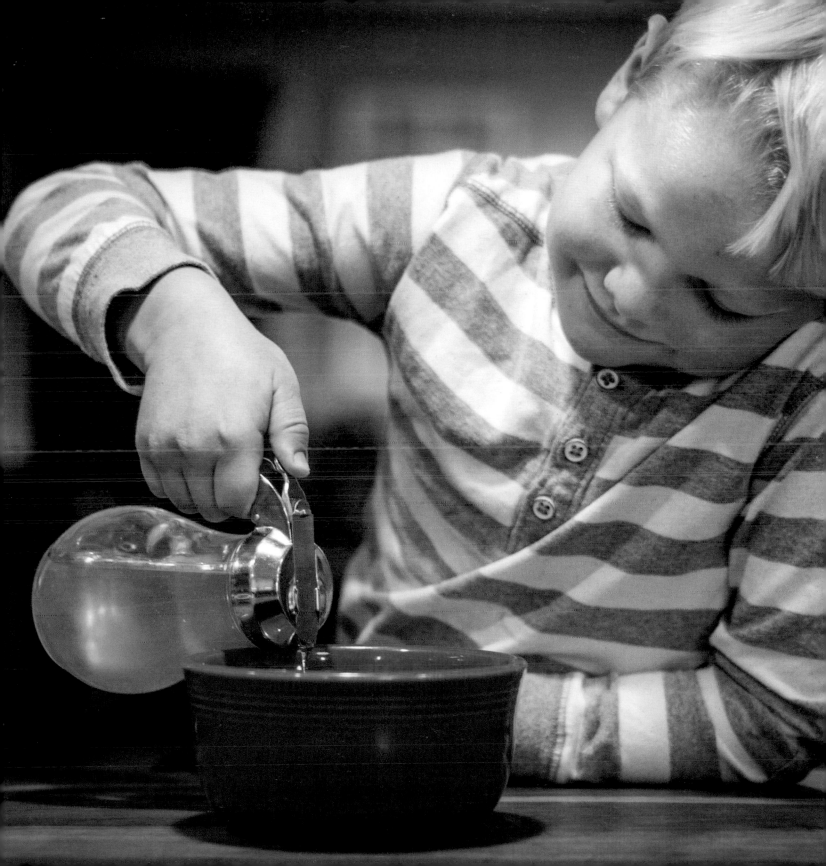

Flower Crowns

Braided flower crowns are easier—and more fun—to make than you might think. And when you wear one, you'll feel like garden or woodland royalty! Made from flexible twigs, flowers, or leaves that you braid together using the technique below, each season offers new crown-making inspiration. Let the forest festival begin!

- An armful of freshly picked herbs or flowers with long, flexible stems
- A few inches of floral wire, yarn, or metal twist-ties

Instructions

1. Begin with three sprigs of your chosen herbs or flowers. Lay them close together and parallel on your work surface.

2. Gently braid them for two or three repeats.

3. Lay a fourth sprig over the top of your braid and join its stem with the shortest of your three original plants.

4. Continue to add new sprigs every inch or two, or as needed, by laying them on top of your work and joining their stems with another in the braid. The shorter your stems, the more often you will have to add new sprigs.

5. Wrap the flower garland around your head to check for length, holding the loose end tightly to ensure it does not unravel.

6. When your flower or herb braid is long enough to reach around your head with a few inches of overlap, use a small piece of floral wire to secure the end, in the same manner you would apply a hair tie to braided hair.

7. Use several small pieces of floral wire to secure the tail behind the decorative braid, forming a crown.

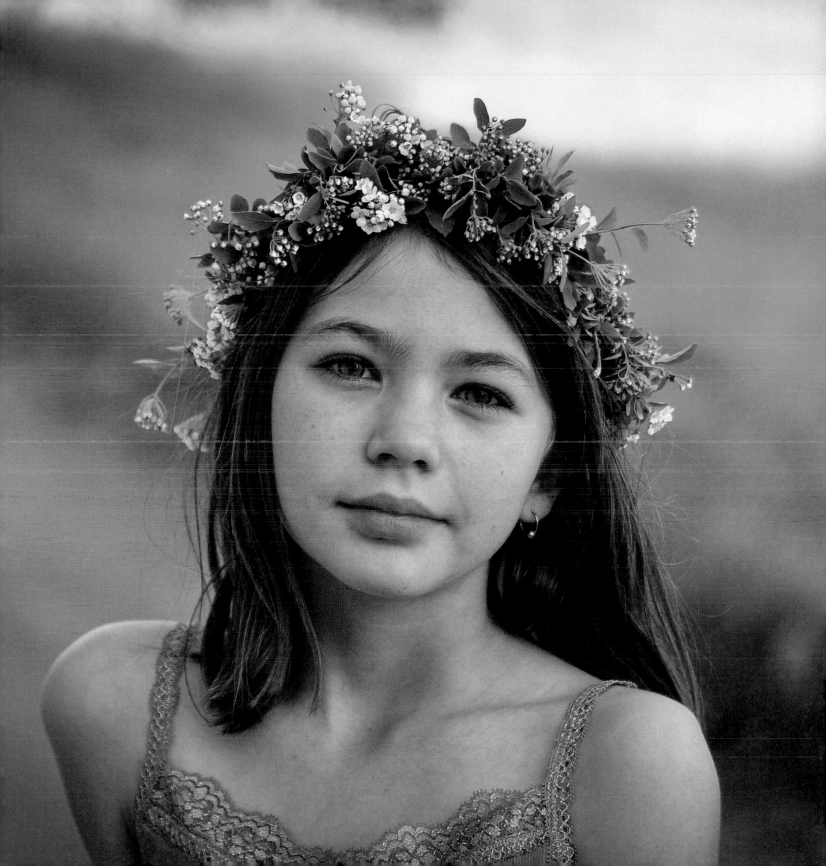

Sunshine Shrub

What on earth is a shrub? No, I don't mean a small tree or bush! "Shrub" is just a funny, old-fashioned name for a refreshing summer drink. Traditionally made of fruit, vinegar, and sugar, this one has dandelion root, raw honey, and probiotic apple cider vinegar. What results is a fruity, tart, syrup to add to fizzy water. This lip-smacking fizzy drink quenches your thirst like nothing else. Healthy *and* delicious? Sign me up!

ACTIVE TIME: Less than 15 minutes, not including foraging and drying time
TOTAL TIME: 10 days | **YIELD:** 3 cups

INGREDIENTS

- ½ cup fresh or frozen raspberries
- 1 cup pitted and chopped fresh or frozen peaches
- Zest and juice of 1 lemon
- ⅓ cup chopped fresh dandelion root, or 3 tablespoons dried
- 1 tablespoon fresh, grated gingerroot
- ½ teaspoon cardamom seeds
- 1½ cups raw apple cider vinegar
- ¾ cup honey
- ¼ cup maple syrup

Instructions

1. Place the peaches, raspberries, lemon zest, and lemon juice in a glass quart-size jar.

2. Muddle the fruit with the back of a wooden spoon, pressing gently to release some juices.

3. Add the dandelion root, ginger, and cardamom. Stir to combine.

4. Add the vinegar, honey, and maple syrup. Stir to dissolve the honey.

5. Cover with a tight-fitting plastic lid or line a metal lid with a piece of a waxed paper, parchment, or a small plastic bag and place in the refrigerator for 10 days, shaking or stirring daily.

6. Strain your shrub through a fine-mesh strainer, gently pressing to extract any extra juice. Transfer to a clean, dry glass bottle or jar. Lid and label.

To use

Add 1 tablespoon Sunshine Shrub concentrate to 8 ounces of carbonated water. Serve chilled or on ice. Adjust the ratios of shrub to water to taste.

Storage

Stored in the refrigerator, homemade shrubs will keep for up to 6 months.

Customize!

If peaches and raspberries are out of season, substitute with plums, pears, or persimmons! Since shrubs are infinitely customizable, you can experiment with any favorite herb and fruit combinations, such as watermelon-mint or strawberry-basil. For a different flavor, replace ¼ cup of the apple cider vinegar with balsamic. Delicious!

Use with caution if any of the following conditions apply:

- Pregnancy
- Kidney stones
- Acid reflux
- Ulcers
- Gallbladder disease or gallstones

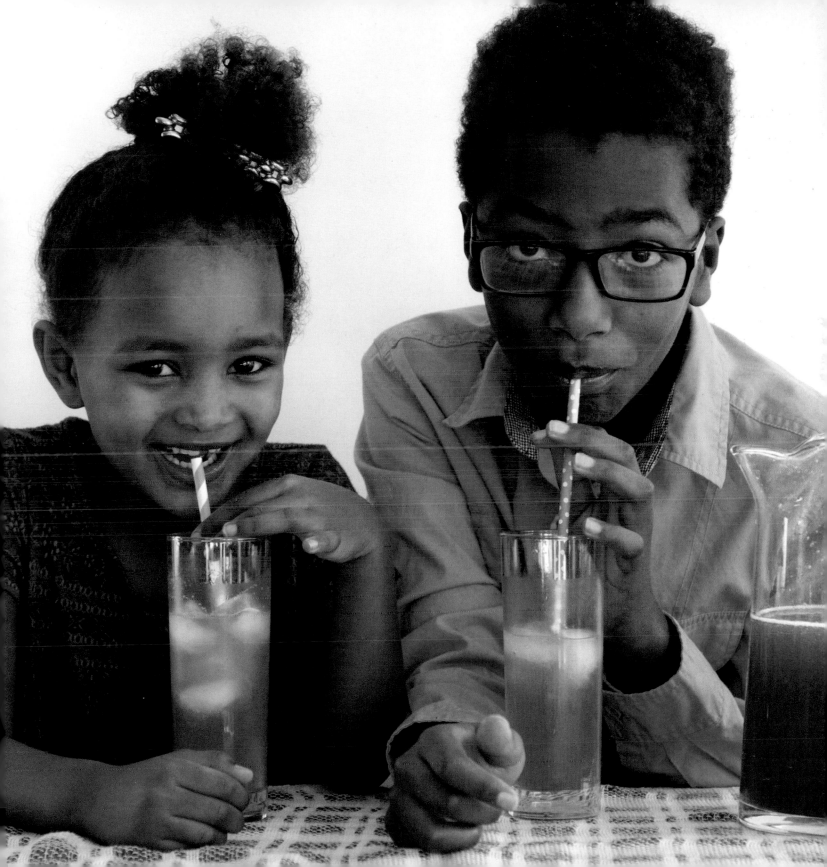

Dandy Dressing

Our dandelion-leaf-infused salad dressing is a tasty way to enjoy the goodness of dandelion without the bitter bite. This delicious dressing might just make salad your favorite part of the meal!

ACTIVE TIME: Less than 15 minutes, not including foraging and wilting or drying time
TOTAL TIME: 4 weeks | **YIELD:** 1 cup

STEP 1: INFUSE YOUR VINEGAR

This delightful dressing begins with dandelion-leaf-infused vinegar. Here's how to make it!

INGREDIENTS

- ½ cup fresh, chopped, wilted dandelion leaf, or a scant ¼ cup dried
- ¾ cup raw apple cider vinegar

Instructions

1. If you're using fresh dandelions, harvest them after the morning dew has dried. Pick over your leaves and remove any debris. Allow to wilt for 12 to 24 hours to reduce moisture.

2. Coarsely chop your wilted dandelion leaves and transfer to a half-pint glass jar.

3. Cover with vinegar and poke it with a chopstick or table knife to release air bubbles. Make sure you add enough vinegar to cover your herbs by a minimum of 1 inch above the plant matter to prevent mold growth.

4. If your herbs float, weigh them down with a clean, dry stone or smaller glass jar placed inside your jar.

5. Cover with a plastic lid or line a metal lid with a piece of a waxed paper, parchment, or a small plastic bag and place it on a plate in an out-of-the-way, shaded corner of the kitchen. Remove the weight and shake your jar daily, or anytime you think of it, always checking that the herbs are completely covered with vinegar after each shake.

6. After 3 to 4 weeks, strain the vinegar through a fine-mesh strainer. Squeeze to extract as much syrup from the leaves as possible. Compost or discard the solids.

7. Transfer the vinegar to a labeled glass jar and store for up to 1 year in a cool, dark place. Or use immediately in the recipe that follows.

STEP 2: MAKE YOUR DRESSING

Once your vinegar is ready, it's time to make your salad dressing.

INGREDIENTS

- ¼ cup dandelion vinegar
- 1½ tablespoons balsamic vinegar
- ½ cup plus 2 tablespoons olive oil
- ½ clove of garlic, minced
- Generous pinch of salt
- A few grinds of black pepper
- 2 tablespoons maple syrup
- 1 scant teaspoon dried thyme

Instructions

1. Place the dressing ingredients in a pint-sized mason jar. Cover the jar with a tight-fitting lid and shake well to combine.

2. Serve on your favorite fresh or wilted greens. Stored covered in the refrigerator, dressing will keep for up to 4 weeks.

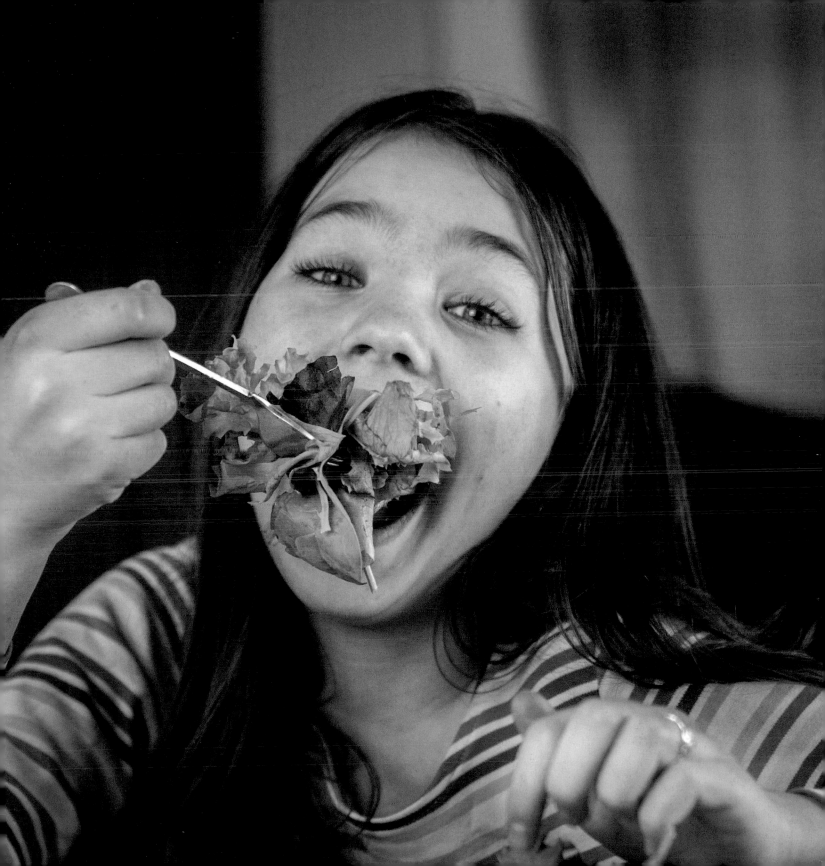

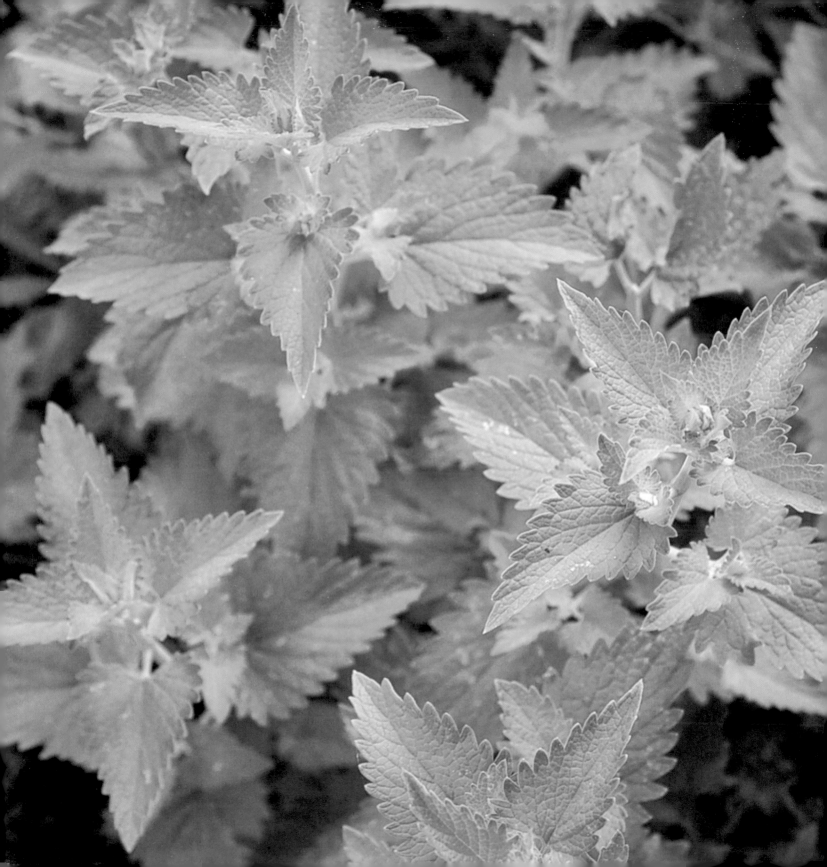

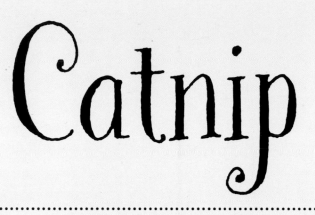

6 Catnip

Oh, hello . . . have we met? I'm Catnip. Perhaps you've heard of me already. You might be familiar with the curious effect I have on cats, causing them to act a little wild. (That's what most people know about me.) Even my scientific name, *Nepeta cataria*, has the word "cat" tucked away inside because of how much cats adore me.

But don't be fooled! While I cause cats to feel frisky, I have the opposite effect on humans. I'm a calming remedy for people, especially for kids.

As a relaxing herb, I am helpful for both cranky days and restless nights. I'm also a nice treatment for upset stomachs and constipation. But I really shine when used for teething discomfort in babies and kids. What a helpful friend I can be!

My nickname, "catmint," is one hint that I belong to the mint family. (Perhaps you've already met my spunkier cousins, peppermint and spearmint.) Other clues that I'm a mint are my square stems and opposite (paired) leaves.

Like other members of the mint family, I am a hardy perennial. Once you plant me, you'll have a steady supply of catnip for years to come. I love the sunshine and enjoy sinking

Latin Name:

Nepeta cataria

Parts Used:
leaves and flowers

Energetics:
cool and dry

Catnip is a helpful herb for:
- Fussy days
- Restless nights
- Stress and anxiety
- Colic
- Constipation
- Upset stomach
- Teething discomfort

my roots into well-drained soil. But be warned: once established, I am hard to remove if you decide to transplant me to a different location! Consider planting me in a clay pot sunken partially into the soil if you'd like to contain my spread.

I am a common volunteer (some might say "weed") in sunny fields and farmyards, so if you live in a rural area you may already have me around.

Though other mints are delicious, I am quite bitter so most people don't appreciate my flavor when used alone. Try blending me with tastier herbs—such as my cousins, peppermint, spearmint, and lemon balm—or with other relaxing (but palatable) herbs, such as chamomile and lavender.

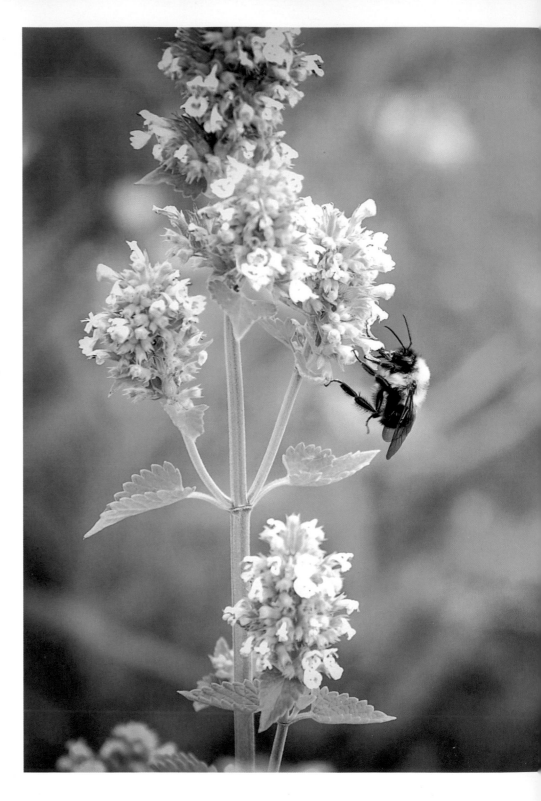

HERBAL ADVENTURES

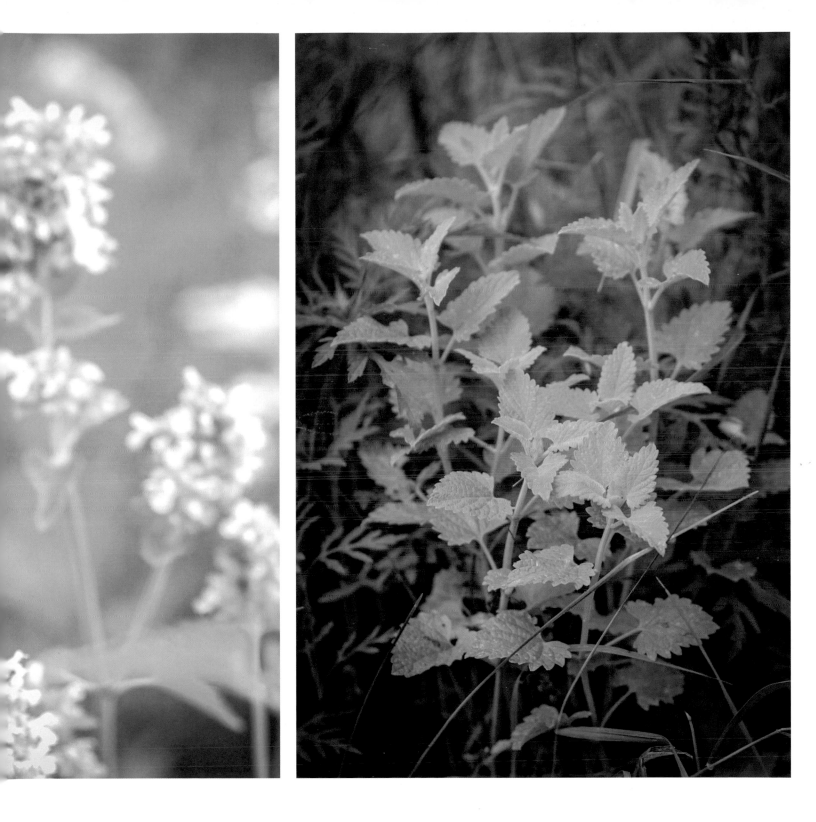

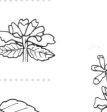
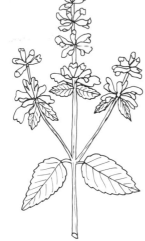

Field Identification

To identify catnip in the field, look for its key distinguishing characteristics. (Use the photograph on the right as a guide.)

Stem:
Catnip (like all members of the mint family) has an erect (upright), square stem. Stems are brittle and easily broken by hand.

Leaves:
Catnip leaves are 1 to 2 inches across, heart-shaped, and deeply lobed, with rounded teeth. The surface of the catnip plant is covered in soft, fuzzy hairs. Up close it almost looks downy. Leaves emerge in pairs that are opposite one another along the stem.

Flowers:
Catnip flowers are white to lavender in color (some with purple spots). Examined close-up, they look like tiny snapdragon flowers. These flowers are arranged in oblong clusters at the top of each stem, with each cluster bearing douncesens of tiny blossoms. Often, you find them buzzing with happy bees, collecting the catnip nectar. Flowers develop midsummer and bloom through the fall.

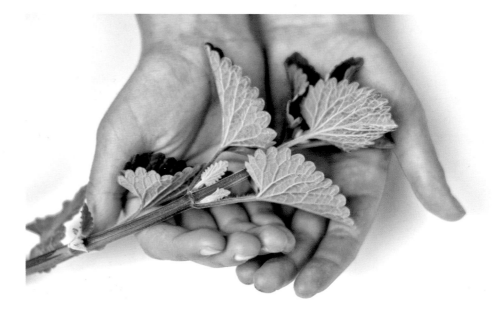

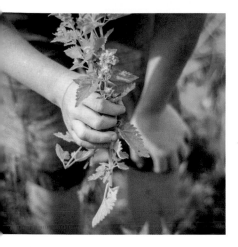

Scent:
The scent of catnip leaves is distinctive. Green, warm, and subtly minty, though less spicy-sweet than other members of the same family.

Growth habit:
Catnip produces multiple stems from the same base. Catnip can grow to 4 feet tall.

Habitat:
Catnip prefers well-drained soil in full or partial sun. Find catnip growing wild in overgrown farmyards, open fields, or empty lots.

Range:
Catnip grows wild throughout most of North America, except in the farthest regions to the north and south.

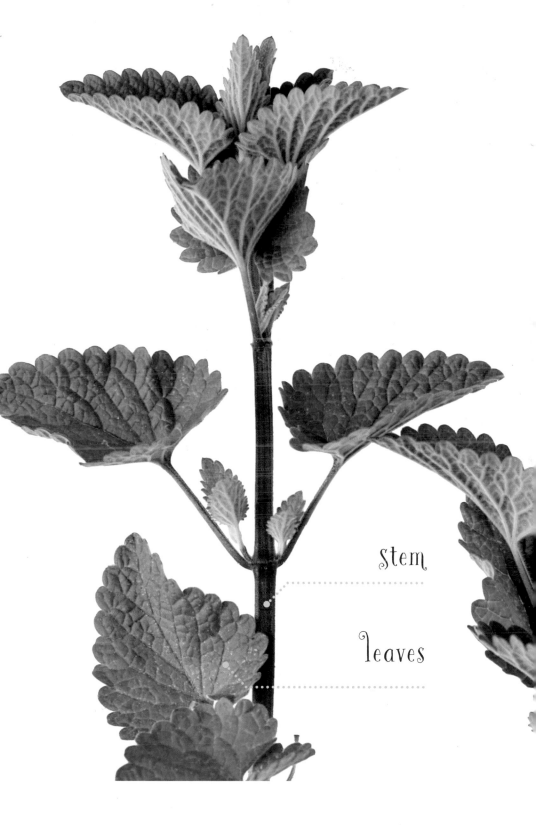

stem

leaves

Calm Kids Tea Blend

INGREDIENTS

- 4 tablespoons dried catnip leaf
- 3 tablespoons dried lemon balm
- 3 tablespoons dried chamomile
- 3 tablespoons dried peppermint
- 2 tablespoons fennel seeds
- 1 tablespoon licorice root
- 1 tablespoon dried rose hips

Catnip and kids were made for each other! Sip a mug-full anytime you need a little calming catnip magic: before a test, when you're overtired, or if you're bouncing off the walls! It's a healthy and safe way to unwind.

TIME: Less than 10 minutes, not including foraging and drying time | **YIELD:** 1 cup dry tea blend

Instructions

1. Measure all ingredients into a clean, dry jar.
2. Crush any large leaves between your fingers if necessary.
3. Cover and shake to combine.
4. Clearly label with tea blend and date for storage.

Not for use during pregnancy.

To use

To brew, measure 1 tablespoon of tea blend into a tea strainer or directly into a teapot. Pour 2 cups of just-boiled water over the tea, and then cover and steep for 5 to 10 minutes. Strain, cool, and serve. If you like, add a drop of honey. Avoid honey for children under one year of age.

Storage

Kept in a cool, dry place, Calm Kids Tea Blend will keep for up to 1 year.

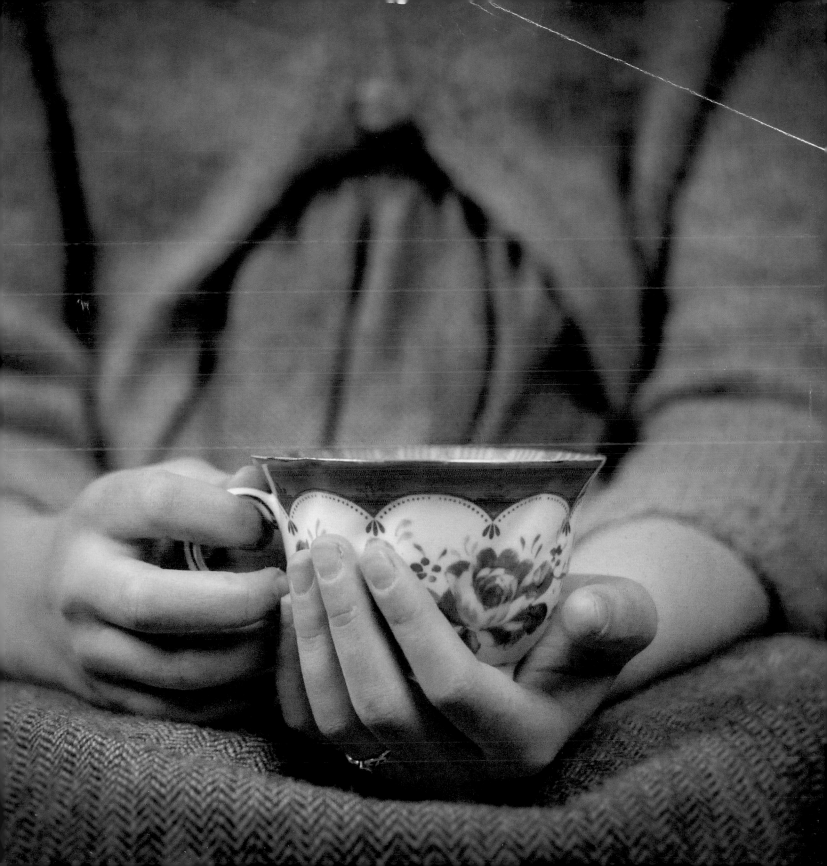

The Young Herbalist's Plant Press

Pressed leaves and flowers are beautiful! They can be used for nature study, art projects, and more. When properly dried and glued to paper alongside some botanical notes, these pressed specimens can become the foundation for a personal herbarium, or dried herb collection. Or get artistic and add them to decorative paper or hand-drawn illustrations. The choice is yours! (Pressed plants are also be used to decorate the paper dolls on page 137.)

(Pressed plants are also be used to decorate the paper dolls on page 137.)

SUPPLIES

- 2 ½×4×6-inch wooden boards, or any size you desire
- Sandpaper (optional)
- Cardboard (for spacers between plants)
- Watercolor paper or office paper (to absorb moisture from drying plants)
- 2 1-inch-wide hook and loop straps, 18 inches long (for a 4×6-inch press)

NOTE: *If you don't have access to woodworking tools, have your pieces pre-cut for you at the lumberyard. If your lumberyard doesn't stock ½-inch boards, check in the trim and baseboards department for wood of a comparable thickness. Or, to simplify the project even more, purchase pre-made plaques from the craft store or cutting boards from a kitchen supply store instead.*

While flowers and leaves can be successfully pressed between the pages of heavy books, a plant press is more convenient. You can even carry it with you into the field and press plants immediately after harvest.

Instructions

Building your own press is easier than you think. I created the plant press shown here with two ½x4x6-inch boards. You can make yours in any size you wish. Try making one small enough for a coat pocket or as big as you can comfortably hold.

Make your plant press.

1. If the boards are rough, sand until smooth with sandpaper.

2. Cut 10 pieces of cardboard down to 3½×5½ inches, or ½ inch smaller than your boards.

3. Cut 18 pieces of watercolor or office paper to the same size as the cardboard.

4. Layer the cardboard and watercolor paper, 1 piece of cardboard, 2 pieces of watercolor paper, until the entire stack is used. Finish with a final piece of cardboard.

5. Place this stack of cardboard and paper between your two boards, and then secure with hook and loop straps.

Press some plants!

6. To use your plant press, harvest on a dry day, after the dew has evaporated. Choose flowers and other plant material that is thin enough to press flat, and avoid large or thick items, such as seedpods and thick blooms or stems. Brush off any dirt or debris and arrange your specimens in a single layer on a piece of watercolor paper. Carefully arrange them to prevent unexpected creases or overlap.

7. When you are satisfied with your placement, cover with a second piece of watercolor paper and top this "sandwich" with another layer of cardboard in your plant press.

8. Secure the hook and loop straps as tightly as you can, and allow the plants to dry for 2 to 3 weeks. Thicker flowers may require additional time.

9. When your plants are completely dry, carefully remove the top sheet of watercolor paper and gently remove your flowers and herbs. They will be brittle, so be gentle with them!

10. Use your pressed plants however you desire.

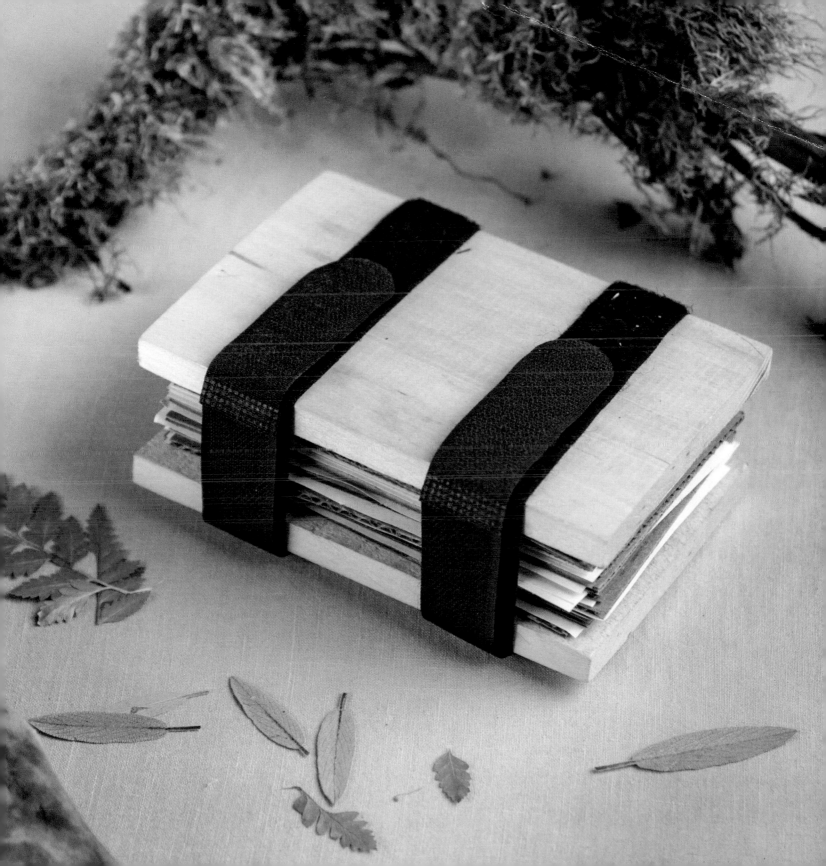

Freezer Teethers

Cutting teeth is no fun for anyone. Bring comfort to your favorite little teether with this comforting, iced remedy. It works like magic! I promise.

TIME: Less than 10 minutes, not including foraging and drying time
YIELD: ½ cup dry tea blend

INGREDIENTS

- 4 tablespoons dried catnip leaf
- 2 tablespoons dried chamomile
- 2 tablespoons dried peppermint

Instructions

1. Measure all ingredients into a clean, dry jar.
2. Crush any large leaves between your fingers if necessary.
3. Cover and shake to combine.
4. Clearly label with tea blend and date for storage.

To use

Measure 1 tablespoon of tea blend into a tea strainer or directly into a teapot. Pour 2 cups of just-boiled water over the tea, and then cover and steep for 5 to 10 minutes. Strain and cool to room temperature. When tea has cooled, soak a clean dry cotton cloth (a washcloth works well) into the brewed tea. Twist the cloth into itself (using a wringing motion) and freeze until solid. Offer a frozen cloth to teething babies and toddlers as needed. Relief!

Storage

Kept in a cool, dry place, the Freezer Teethers tea blend will keep for up to 1 year.

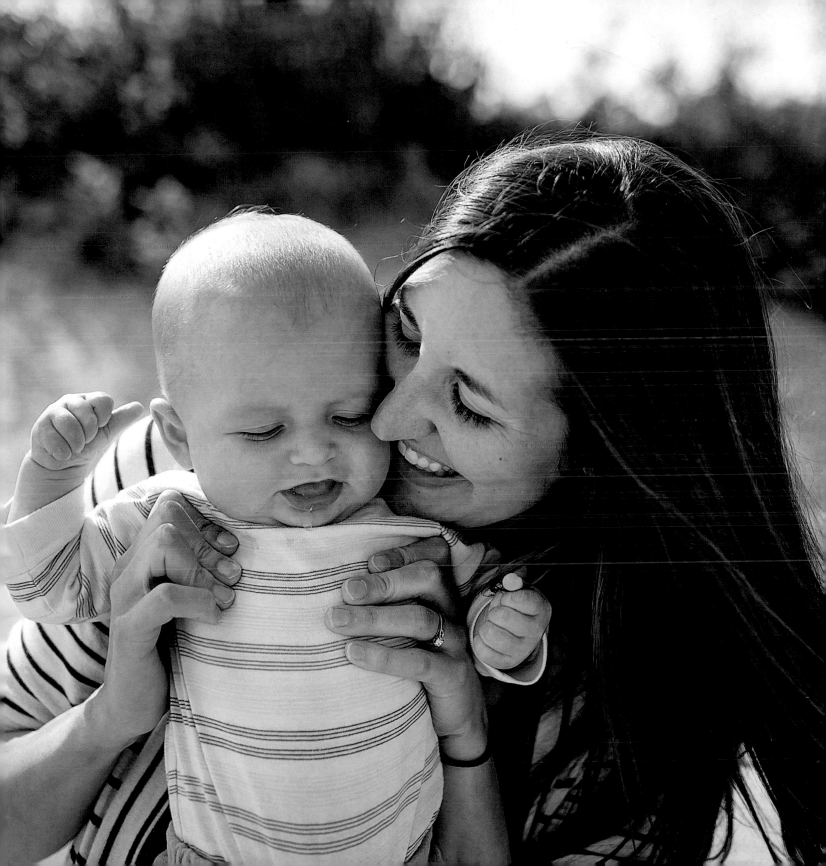

Catnip Glycerite

No time for tea? Glycerites are a sweet and tasty option when you need a remedy in a hurry. Catnip glycerite is as soothing as its freshly brewed cousin, catnip tea. We like to have some handy for nights when we can't fall asleep, or times we're anxious or agitated. Keep a bottle on hand for anytime you need calming catnip—quick!

ACTIVE TIME: Less than 10 minutes, not including foraging and wilting or drying time
TOTAL TIME: 4 to 6 weeks | **YIELD:** ¾ cup

INGREDIENTS

- 1½ cups fresh catnip leaf, or ½ cup dried
- ¾ to 1 cup glycerin, depending on method used
- ¼ cup water if using dried catnip

Instructions

1. Using the ingredients listed at left, follow the instructions on pages 166 or 167 to make your choice of a fresh or dried herb glycerite. Choose the appropriate recipe based on the type of catnip you have available available (fresh or dried).

2. Clearly label your finished glycerite with the remedy name and date.

To use

Glycerites may be taken straight or added to a cup of tea. They are also delicious stirred into applesauce.

Not for use during pregnancy.

Dosage

Children may take 1 to 2 drops per 10 pounds of body weight. Adults may take ½ teaspoon up to 5 times per day, as needed.

Storage

Stored in a cool, dry place, Catnip Glycerite will keep for at least 1 year.

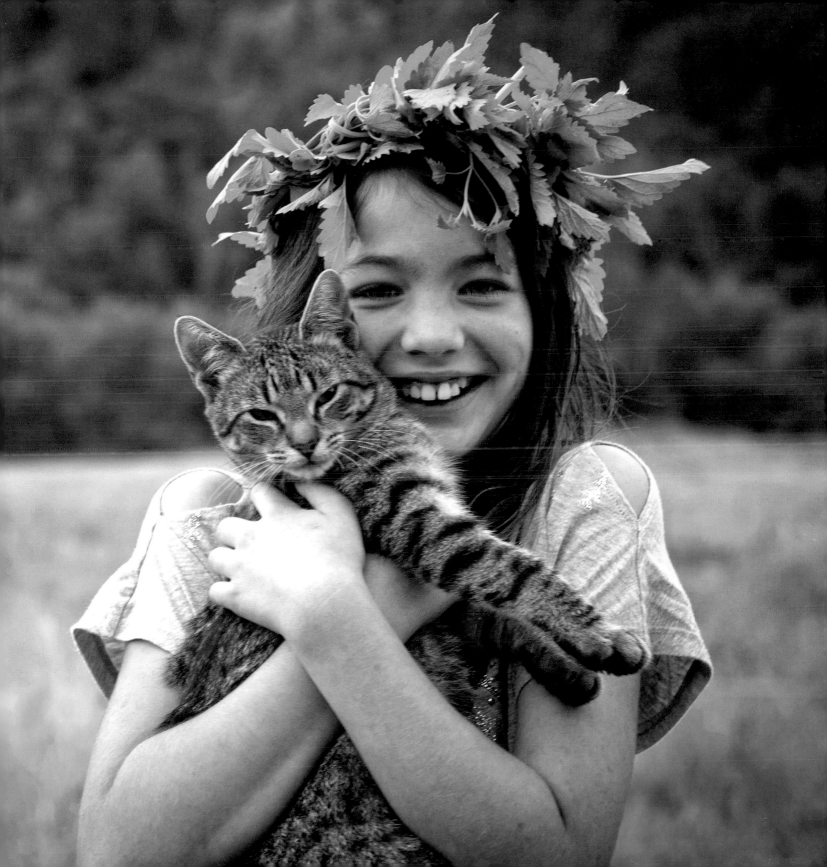

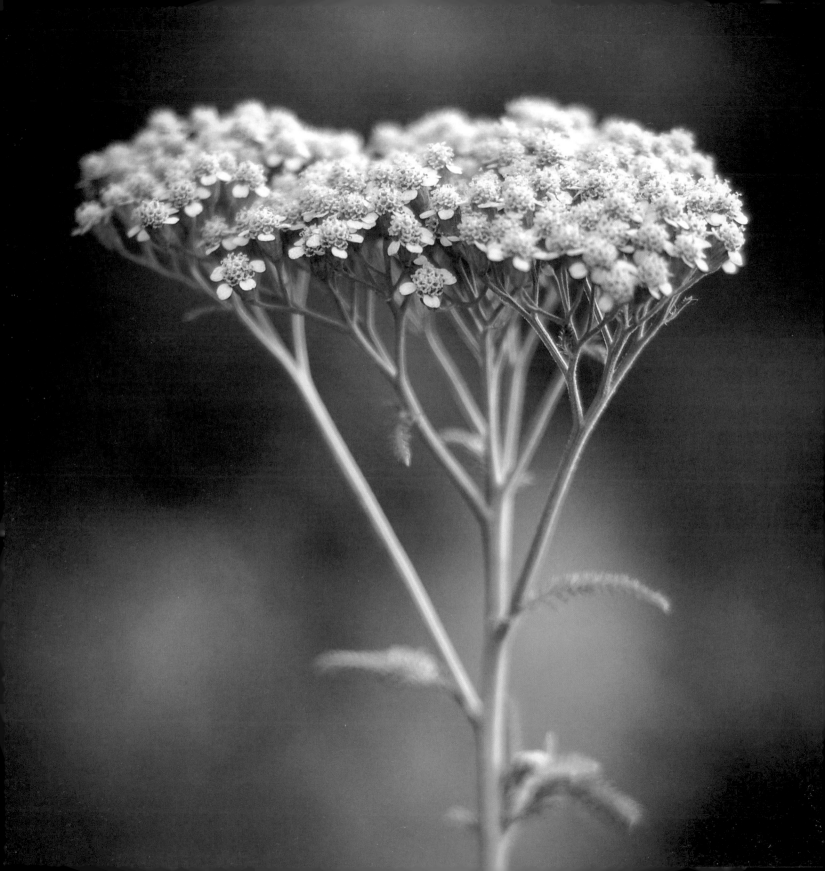

7 Yarrow

Achillea millefolium, reporting for duty! I'm at the ready to assist with all of your first aid needs. Cuts, scrapes, nosebleeds, fevers, stomachaches—I'm here to tend to them all! Just tell me what needs attention first.

I'm sorry—I've gotten ahead of myself. We haven't yet properly met. Most people call me yarrow. My Latin name, *Achillea*, is taken from the Greek hero Achilles. Perhaps I was the herb that Achilles used to heal his soldiers on the battlefield. I'd like to think so, since I'm well-suited for the job. Indeed, my nickname, "soldier's woundwort," is a nod to this historic use.

While garden varieties of yarrow come in a rainbow of colors, they are known more for their looks than their medicine. My flowers, on the other hand, are a no-nonsense cream color.

As an antiseptic and anti-inflammatory herb, I'm a great choice for stopping bleeding—cuts, scrapes, even nosebleeds. I can also help to quickly reduce swelling from strains and sprains. But there's more that I can do! Reach for me to reduce a fever, stimulate digestion, and soothe an upset stomach. What else can I help with? More conditions that I have time to list. (My nickname "cure-all" was nobly earned.) Now then. What needs tending first?

Latin Name:

Achillea millefolium

Parts Used:
leaves and flowers

Energetics:
complex (can be both warm and cool, and dry and damp)

Yarrow is a helpful herb for:
- Speeding healing of cuts and scrapes
- Soothing sprains and strains
- Stimulating sluggish digestion
- Cooling fevers
- Relieving stomach cramps

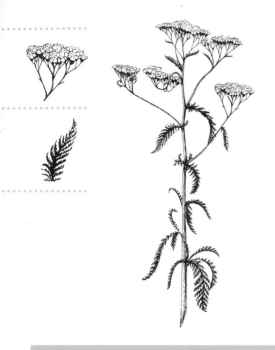

Field Identification

To identify yarrow in the field, look for its key distinguishing characteristics. (Use the photograph on the right as a guide.)

Stem:
Yarrow's stem is sturdy, dry, and almost woody. It is sparsely covered in alternately arranged delicate, feathery leaves.

Leaves:
Yarrow leaves are long and lance-shaped. They are deeply divided, giving them a soft, feathery, fern-like appearance. They are arranged alternately along the stem and become noticeably smaller as they grow from the ground toward the flower head. The leaves that surround the base of stem are much larger than those on the stem itself.

Flowers:
Yarrow flowers emerge in clusters at the tip of each stem. They are dull or creamy off-white in color. Each flower has four to six petals, which are notched at the tip. These petals surround a cluster of pastel yellow disc florets. (On rare occasions, wild yarrow can be found with soft pink flowers instead of the usual off-white.)

- Not for internal use during pregnancy.

- Not for use by people with allergies to the *Compositae* family.

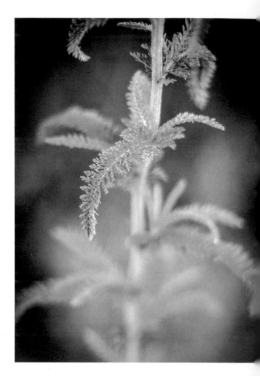

Stem:
Yarrow grows 1 to 3 feet tall on a solid branching stem. The stem is slightly textured, with an almost scratchy covering of short, fine hairs.

Scent:
Yarrow leaves and flowers bear a pleasant savory-spicy aroma, not unlike a combination of several culinary herbs including rosemary and oregano.

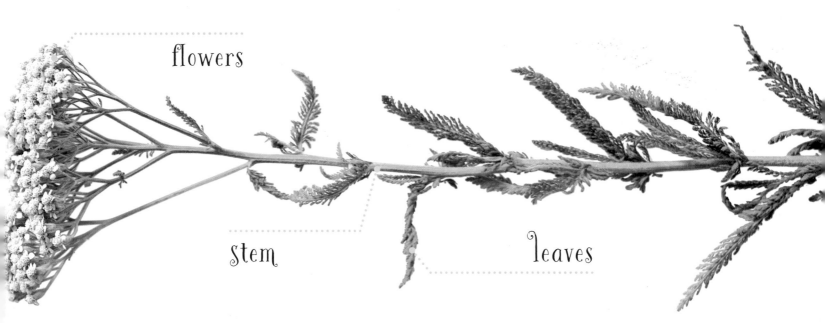

flowers

stem

leaves

Lookalikes

Yarrow has two potential lookalikes: Queen Anne's lace (or wild carrot) and deadly water hemlock. While Queen Anne's lace is an edible and medicinal plant in its own right, water hemlock is poisonous and must be avoided.

To determine if you have *truly* found yarrow, take the time to carefully examine the leaves, stem, flowers, and root.

Stems and Leaves:
Water hemlock stems are hairless and hollow, as opposed to yarrow's hairy, solid stems. Water hemlock leaves are shiny and resemble fern leaflets, while yarrow leaves are soft and feathery.

Flowers:
Yarrow flowers grow in a flat-topped cluster of creamy white blossoms. Both Queen Anne's lace and water hemlock grow in larger umbrella-shaped flower heads.

Root:
Both Queen Anne's lace and water hemlock grow from a sturdy taproot. If you are still unsure, confirm that you have yarrow by taking a look at the roots. Because yarrow grows from spreading rhizomes, this final characteristic will let you know that you have found the right plant.

Growth habit:
Yarrow grows approximately 2 feet tall, emerging in clusters from the ground. The stems are normally encircled by a group of longer leaves at the base. Each stem divides toward the top into a unified cluster of flowers.

Habitat:
Yarrow thrives in full or partial sun and is commonly found in grasslands, forest edges, and alongside country lanes.

Range:
Yarrow is found throughout all of North America and much of Europe.

Cuts and Scrapes Oil

INGREDIENTS

- ¼ cup dried yarrow leaf, or ½ cup fresh
- ¼ cup dried calendula flowers, or ¾ cup fresh, wilted and chopped
- 1 cup olive oil, or other neutral oil

Skinned knees and shallow cuts don't stand a chance! Yarrow-infused oil is just the thing to quiet pain, speed healing, and reduce the chance of a scar. One of my favorite herbal remedies, a small bottle of it is always in my first aid kit.

ACTIVE TIME: Less than 10 minutes, not including foraging and drying time
TOTAL TIME: 1 day to 4 weeks, depending on infusion method | **YIELD:** 1 scant cup

Instructions

1. Using the ingredients listed above, follow the instructions on pages 169 or 170 to create your infused oil. Choose whichever method you prefer: solar or stovetop.

2. Be sure to clearly label your finished oil with the infusion type and date.

To use

Apply Cuts and Scrapes Oil to any superficially injured skin. Cover with gauze or a bandage and reapply as needed.

Storage

Stored in a cool dry place, Cuts and Scrapes Oil should last up to 1 year.

Not for use on puncture wounds or very deep cuts until after the wound has begun to heal.

Variation: Cuts and Scrapes Balm

Use your infused oil to create a balm, following the instructions on page 48.

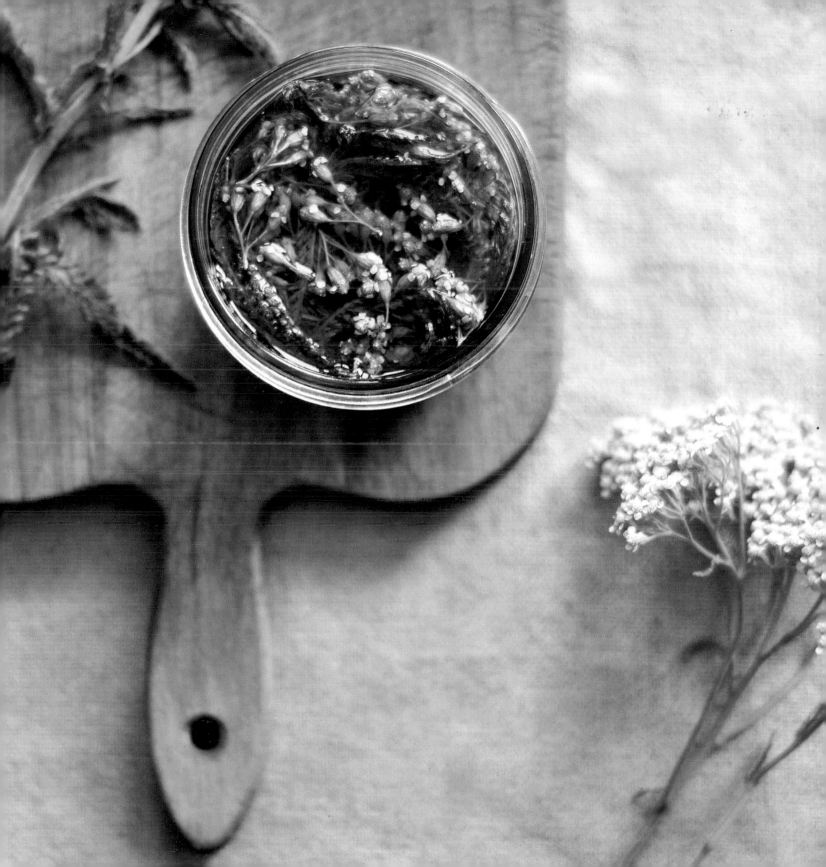

Bumps and Bruises Wound Wash

A wonderful remedy for scraped, bruised skin resulting from a hard tumble, this infusion is meant for gently cleaning tender wounds to remove debris and promote healing.

TIME: Less than 30 minutes, not including foraging and drying time
YIELD: Approximately 1½ cups

INGREDIENTS

- ½ cup fresh, chopped yarrow leaf and flower, or scant ¼ cup dried
- 3 tablespoons fresh or dried calendula flowers (optional)
- 2 cups water

Instructions

1. Place the yarrow and optional calendula in a small glass or stainless steel pot.

2. Cover with the water and place over medium-high heat. Cover and bring to a simmer.

3. Remove from heat and steep until warm to the touch, approximately 20 minutes.

4. Strain your warm infusion through a fine-mesh strainer lined with a thin cotton towel or a few layers of cheesecloth. Gently press your herbs to extract as much liquid as possible. Discard the solids.

To use

Dip a clean, soft cloth into the infusion until saturated. Wring out slightly and clean the injury using a gentle touch. Alternately, the affected area can be soaked in a basin of the infusion for 2 to 3 minutes. Repeat as desired to ease discomfort and speed healing. Discard any leftover infusion, making a fresh batch for each application.

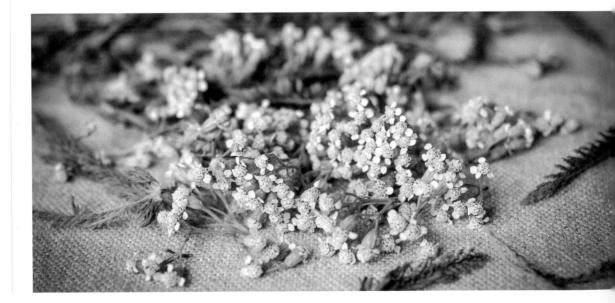

- 2 tablespoons dried yarrow flowers and leaves
- 2 tablespoons dried peppermint leaf
- 2 tablespoons dried elderflowers
- 1 teaspoon dried licorice root
- 1 teaspoon dried rose hips
- 1 teaspoon dried spearmint

Romani Flu and Fever Tea

Legend says that a recipe for yarrow, peppermint, and elder tea (for fevers, flus, and colds) has been passed down by countless generations of European Romani. My version includes other helpful herbs as well, while honoring the roots of this classic blend.

TIME: Less than 10 minutes, not including foraging and drying time
YIELD: ½ scant cup dry tea blend

Instructions

1. Measure all the ingredients into a clean, dry mixing bowl.

2. Crush any large leaves between your fingers if necessary, and stir well to combine.

3. Transfer to a clean glass jar.

4. Lid and label.

Not for use during pregnancy.

To use

To brew, set a kettle of fresh water to boil. Measure 1 tablespoon of tea blend into a tea strainer or directly into a teapot. Pour 2 cups hot water over the tea, and then cover and steep for 10 minutes. Strain, cool, and serve. If you like, add a dash of honey.

Storage

Stored in a cool, dry place, Romani Flu and Fever Tea should last for up to 1 year.

Herbal Rice Buddy

Filled with rice and fragrant dried herbs, then warmed in the oven or microwave, a rice buddy is calming and comforting for all ages. Adults, teens, and young children all seem equally drawn to the comfort and warmth of this simple project.

SUPPLIES

- 100 percent cotton or wool fabric
- Sewing pins
- Sewing needle and sturdy thread
- Sewing machine (optional)
- Chopstick or knitting needle
- Funnel
- ½ to 1 cup dry rice
- 1 tablespoon fragrant dried herbs, crumbled (lavender, yarrow, and catnip are all lovely choices)

Instructions

1. Cut out 2 squares of fabric in any size of your liking. Pictured here are 4-, 5-, and 6-inch rice buddies. The 6-inch is the most popular in our home, but the 4-inch is small enough to fit comfortably in pockets.

2. Place the fabric right sides together and pin to secure.

3. By hand or by machine, sew your rice buddy. Leaving a 2-inch opening at the center of one side, sew with a ½-inch seam allowance all around. This is achieved most easily by beginning your seam 1 inch off-center on one side, and then sewing around in a continuous stitch. End your seam 2 inches from where you began. If machine sewing, backstitch at the beginning and end of your seam to secure.

4. Snip off the corners just outside of the seam, and then turn your pillow right-side out.

5. With a chopstick or knitting needle, push out the corners to form a neat square.

6. Using a funnel, fill the rice buddy until it feels comfortably full (but not stuffed) in your hand. Add the dried herbs.

7. Sew your rice buddy closed with small stitches by hand, and secure with a sturdy knot.

To use

To warm your rice buddy, heat in your choice of an oven or a microwave. Always test the temperature of your rice buddy before giving it to a young child, as they can become quite hot.

Oven heating instructions: Preheat the oven to 250°F with a rack placed in the center. Lay the rice buddies on a clean, dry baking sheet and heat for 20 minutes. Check after 10 minutes, turning the rice buddies over to ensure even heating. The larger the rice buddy, the longer it will take to heat.

Microwave heating instructions: Heat for 15 to 45 seconds, depending on size of the rice buddy. Check every 15 seconds during microwaving until desired heat level is achieved.

Rice buddies will maintain warmth for 10 to 20 minutes, depending on size and heating time.

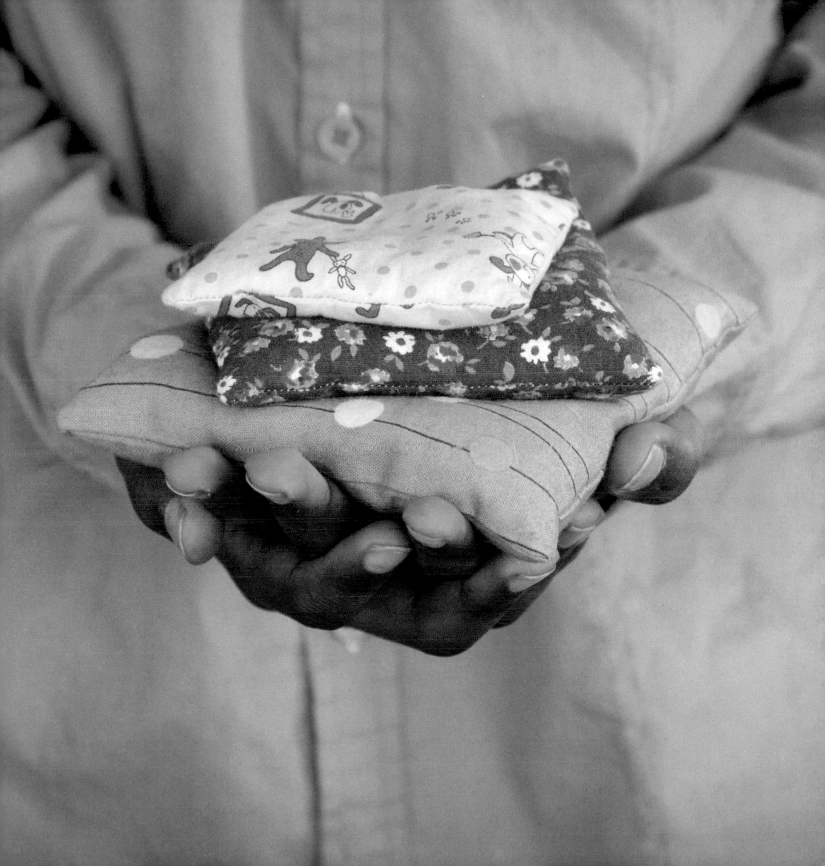

Yarrow Yummy Tummy Tea

INGREDIENTS

- ❀ 2 tablespoons dried yarrow flowers and leaves
- ❀ 2 tablespoons peppermint leaf
- ❀ 2 tablespoons fennel seed
- ❀ 1 tablespoon dried chopped or grated gingerroot
- ❀ 2 teaspoons chopped (cut/sifted) licorice root
- ❀ 2 teaspoons cardamom seeds

This herbal tea blend is helpful for everyday stomach upset. Though yarrow alone is quite bitter, in this tea it's combined with tasty peppermint, ginger, and cardamom for a drink you'll crave even when you don't have a tummy ache! Enjoy before or after meals to encourage healthy digestion.

TIME: Less than 10 minutes, not including foraging and drying time
YIELD: ½ cup dry tea blend

Instructions

1. Measure all the ingredients into a clean, dry mixing bowl.

2. Crush any large leaves between your fingers if necessary and stir well to combine.

3. Transfer to a clean glass jar.

4. Lid and label.

To use

To brew, set a kettle of fresh water to boil. Measure 1 tablespoon of tea blend into a tea strainer or directly into a teapot. Pour 2 cups hot water over the tea, and then cover and steep for 10 minutes. Strain, cool, and serve. If you like, add a dash of honey.

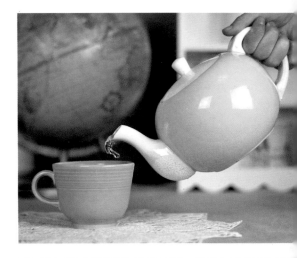

Not for use during pregnancy.

Storage

Stored in a cool, dry place, Yarrow Yummy Tummy Tea should last for up to 1 year.

Yarrow Styptic Powder

A styptic powder helps stop bleeding fast, whether from a cut, a scrape, or even a nosebleed. While some styptics are made with salt (ouch!), I prefer a gentle, but effective, styptic made of powdered yarrow. It couldn't be easier to create, and it's a smart addition to every first aid kit. One pinch sprinkled on a fresh cut or in a nostril with a nosebleed will quickly halt bleeding. Yarrow is also a champion at reducing pain from cuts and abrasions. Because it is antiseptic and anti-inflammatory, yarrow will continue to do good even after the bleeding has stopped.

TIME: Less than 5 minutes, not including foraging and drying time | **YIELD:** 2 tablespoons

Instructions

1. Place the yarrow leaf in a clean, dry coffee grinder or blender.

2. Process until finely powdered, approximately 3 to 4 minutes

3. Transfer to a dry glass jar or metal tin.

4. Lid and label.

To use

Simply sprinkle a pinch of Yarrow Styptic Powder on an injury to stop bleeding. For a bloody nose, place a small pinch inside the nostril or nostrils that are bleeding.

NOTE: *While yarrow styptic powder normally reduces discomfort from cuts and scrapes, in rare cases it can sting when applied. Test on a small part of cut or scrape first before applying throughout.*

Storage

Stored tightly sealed in a cool, dry location, Yarrow Styptic Powder will keep for at least 1 year.

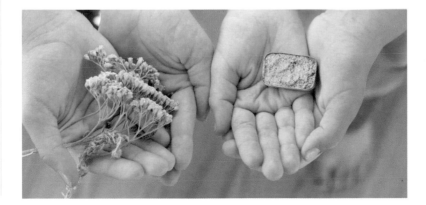

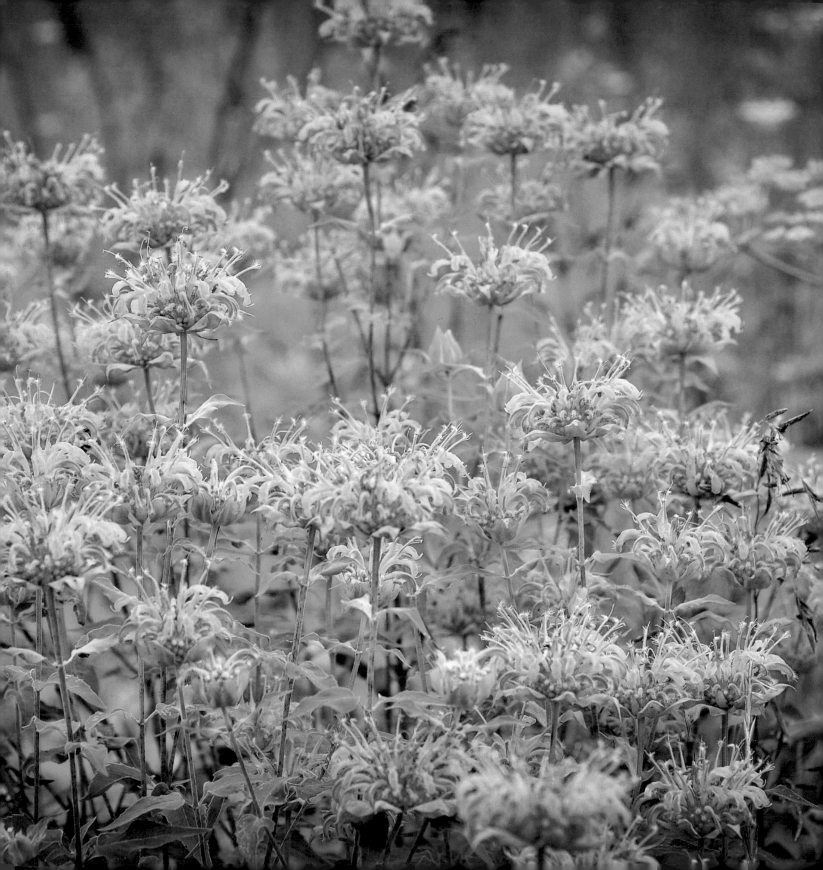

8 Bee Balm

Hello! I'm delighted to meet you, new friend. My name is Monarda—or wild bee balm, if it's easier for you to remember. I'm known by so many names, it's sometimes hard to keep track of them all. While herbalists call me Monarda, the old-timers call me bee balm, wild bergamot, Oswego tea, and sometimes horsemint.

But don't confuse me with the garden varieties of bee balm if you want to use me for soothing sore throats or for treating gassiness, mouth infections, and toothaches. For any of these ailments, only the wild sort (*Monarda fistulosa*, or in a pinch, the wild red-flowered variety, *Monarda didyma*) will yield the results you seek. If you're not sure if the Monarda you've found is a wild variety, crush a leaf between your fingers. I have a very strong smell—similar to fresh thyme or oregano, but a bit spicier and even a little citrusy. If my scent is unimpressive, the recipes you make with me will be unimpressive as well. Keep looking until you find *wild* bee balm growing, well, wild!

I am a member of the mint family, bearing the telltale square stem and opposite (paired) leaves. I love to grow with my face in the sunshine and can often be found growing along the forest edge, on roadsides, in open fields and on prairies.

Latin Name:

Monarda fistulosa

Parts Used:
leaves, flowers, and buds

Energetics:
warm and dry

Bee balm is a helpful herb for:
- Soothing sore throats
- Clearing congestion
- Quieting coughs
- Easing toothaches
- Reducing infections
- Calming burns

119

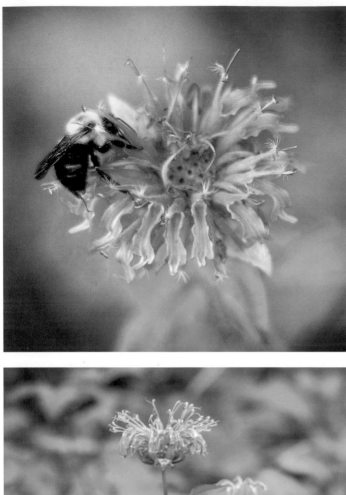

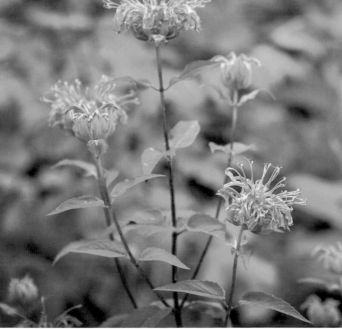

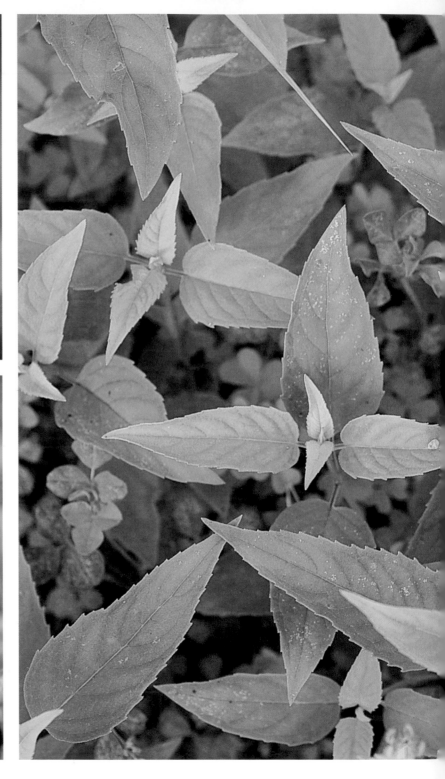

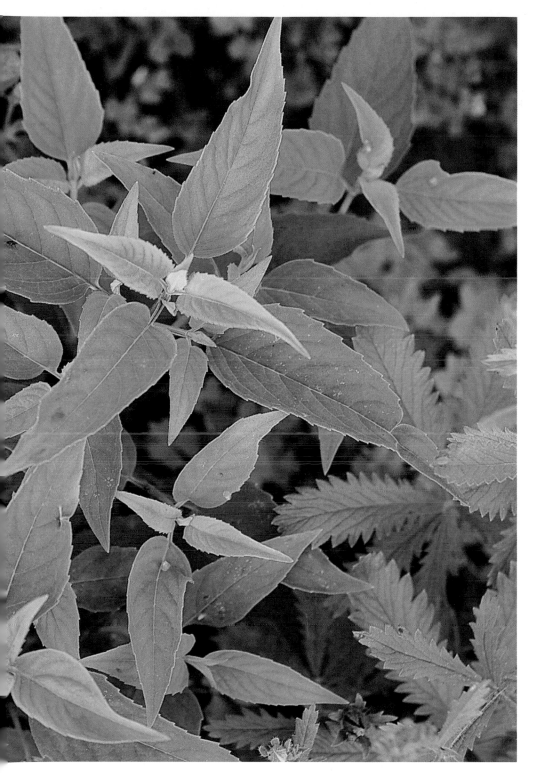

As you may have guessed, I'm called bee balm because I am loved by bees of every sort. My pale-purple, tubular flowers lure them in from miles around, and they delight in sipping my nectar! I bloom beginning in midsummer and finish up just before autumn arrives. When you harvest, be sure to leave plenty of my flowers blooming for the bees too!

I am prone to a white bloom upon my leaves, called powdery mildew. While it won't harm you, make sure the plants you choose are free of these white spots for the highest-quality herbs.

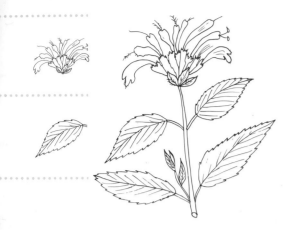

Field Identification

To identify wild bee balm in the field, look for its key distinguishing characteristics. (Use the photograph on the right as a guide.)

Stem:
Like all members of the mint family, bee balm stems are square.

Leaves:
Elongated, lance- or triangle-shaped leaves are arranged in pairs along the stem. Leaves are coarsely toothed. They are slightly hairy on the undersides and smooth on the tops. Powdery mildew is common (especially in damp seasons or shady environments), causing the upper side of the leaf to also appear hairy. Leaves are normally 1 to 2 inches long and 1 inch wide at their widest part, tapering to a point at the distal (far) end.

Flowers:
Lavender-colored flower heads are arranged at the end of each branching stem. They are approximately 1½ inches across and are composite heads comprised of many tubular flowers. The other wild bee balm species, *Monarda didyma*, bears larger red flowers of the same shape.

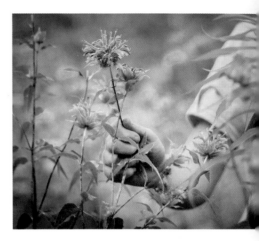

Scent: Wild bee balm smells like a spicy mix of Earl Grey tea, oregano, and thyme. The strongest scent is noticed when crushing a leaf between your fingers.

Growth habit:
Bee balm grows 2 to 4 feet tall in bush-like clusters of many stems.

Habitat:
Bee balm can thrive in slightly dry to slightly moist soil. It is commonly found along the edges of forests, alongside country lanes, and in grasslands.

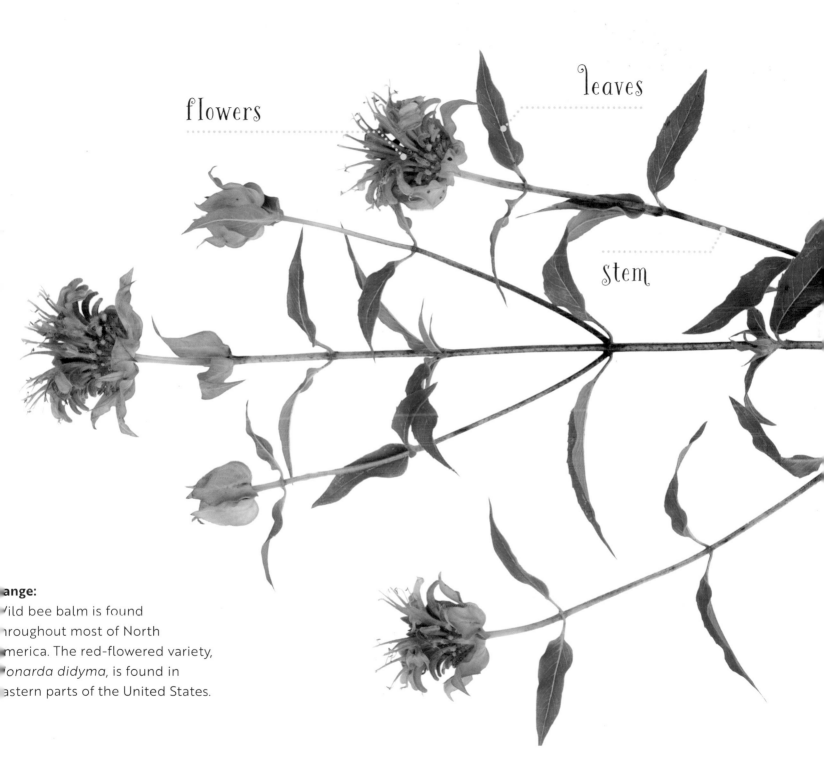

flowers

leaves

stem

ange:
/ild bee balm is found
hroughout most of North
merica. The red-flowered variety,
onarda didyma, is found in
astern parts of the United States.

Throat Soother Oxymel

INGREDIENTS

- 2 cups fresh bee balm leaves and flowers, or 1 cup dried
- ¼ cup fresh sage leaves, or 1½ tablespoon dried
- 2 tablespoons fresh thyme, or 2 teaspoons dried
- ½ cup raw honey
- 1 cup raw apple cider vinegar (labeled "unpasteurized" or "with the mother")

> Talk to your doctor about taking bee balm oxymel if you have a thyroid imbalance. Speak to your care provider regarding use when pregnant. Contains honey. Not for children under one year of age.

In this oxymel, every ingredient is meant to comfort dry, sore, or scratchy throats—from the honey and vinegar to the three herbs. Even if you think you don't like its flavor right away, don't toss it aside! Once you get your first cold of the season, try it again. Chances are it will taste delicious when you need it.

ACTIVE TIME: Less than 10 minutes, not including foraging and wilting or drying time
TOTAL TIME: 4 to 6 weeks | **YIELD:** 1¼ cups

Instructions

1. If using fresh herbs, harvest after the morning dew has dried. Pick them over and remove any garden debris. Pull the bee balm flowers and leaves from the stems, and then allow plants to wilt for 12 to 24 hours to reduce moisture.

2. Coarsely chop the herbs and transfer to a glass pint jar.

3. Cover with the honey and vinegar and poke bee balm mixture with a chopstick or table knife to release air bubbles. If your jar is not completely full, add additional honey or vinegar to fill to the shoulders. Make sure you add enough liquid to cover the herbs by a minimum of ¼ to ½ inch above the plant matter to prevent molding.

4. If your herbs float, weigh them down with a clean, dry stone or smaller glass jar placed inside your pint jar.

5. Lid and label your jar and place it in a dark, out-of-the-way place to infuse.

6. Remove the weight and shake the jar occasionally, pushing the leaves back under the surface if needed after shaking. Add additional honey or vinegar if required to keep your plant material properly submerged.

7. Allow to steep for 4 to 6 weeks, continuing to shake daily or as often as you think of it.

8. After 4 to 6 weeks (or when you feel a cold or sore throat coming on), strain your oxymel. Pour it through a clean, dry piece of cheesecloth, squeezing to extract as much goodness as possible from the herbs. Compost or discard the solids, and transfer the oxymel to a clean, dry glass jar or bottle.

To use

Adults take 1 to 2 teaspoons as needed for sore throat discomfort, up to 8 times per day; children take ½ teaspoon as needed for a sore throat, up to 8 times per day.

Storage

Throat Soother Oxymel will keep for at least 1 year if stored in a cool, dark place.

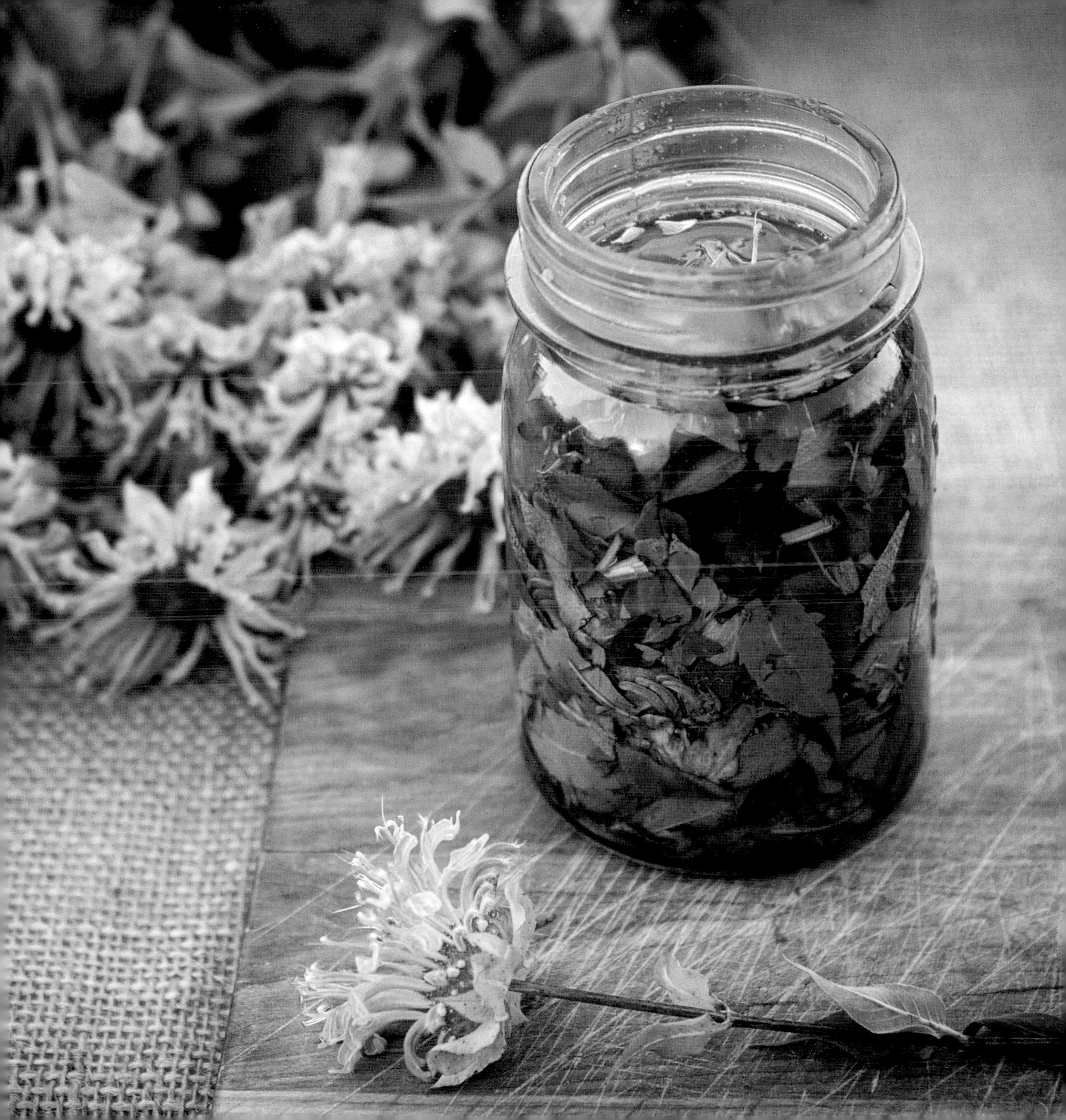

Cold and Flu Season Glycerite

INGREDIENTS

- ½ cup wilted fresh bee balm, or a scant ¼ cup dried
- ½ cup wilted fresh echinacea (a mixture of flower, root, and leaf), or a scant ¼ cup dried
- 2 tablespoons usnea (optional)
- ¾ to 1 cup glycerin, depending on method used

This gentle, kid-friendly remedy is just the thing to help you back on your feet when a cold or flu strikes! Take at the first sign of illness, and then stop taking as soon as you feel like yourself again. I especially love it stirred into a mug of Roman Flu and Fever Tea (page 113)!

ACTIVE TIME: Less than 10 minutes, not including foraging and wilting or drying time
TOTAL TIME: 4 to 6 weeks | **YIELD:** ¾ cup

Instructions

1. Using the ingredients listed above, follow the instructions on pages 166 or 167 to make your choice of a fresh or dried herb glycerite.

2. Clearly label your finished glycerite with the remedy name and date.

To use

At the first sign of a cold or flu take a dose every 4 hours until your symptoms begin to subside. Glycerites may be taken straight or added to a cup of tea. They are also delicious stirred into applesauce.

Dosage

At the first sign of a cold or flu take one dose every 3 to 4 hours until your symptoms begin to subside, or for up to 4 days. Children may take ¼ teaspoon per dose; adults may take ½ to 1 teaspoon.

Storage

Stored in a cool, dry place, Cold and Flu Season Glycerite will keep for at least 1 year.

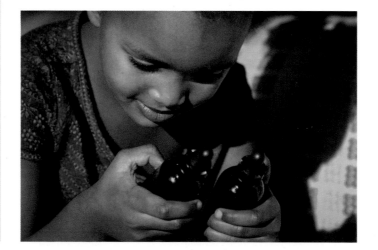

Warm-Me-Up Herbal Tea

INGREDIENTS

- ¼ cup dried bee balm leaves and flowers
- ¼ cup dried holy basil leaves
- 2 tablespoons dried chopped ginger
- 2 tablespoons fennel seeds

This warm and spicy tea is just the thing for a cold winter day. Ginger and bee balm will help warm you up right down to your toes, while fennel and holy basil can soothe stomach upset. Together they can jumpstart slow digestion, soothe a tummy ache, banish gas, and boost your immune system. Not bad for just four ingredients!

TIME: Less than 10 minutes, not including foraging and drying time
YIELD: ¾ cup dry tea blend

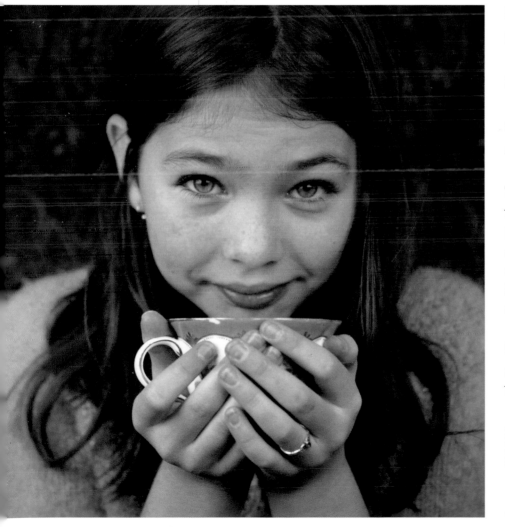

Instructions

1. Measure all ingredients into a clean, dry mixing bowl.

2. Crush any large leaves between your fingers if necessary, and stir well to combine.

3. Transfer to a clean glass jar.

4. Lid and label.

To use

To brew, set a kettle of fresh water to boil. Measure 1 tablespoon of tea blend into a tea strainer or directly into a teapot. Pour 2 cups hot water over the tea, and then cover and steep for 3 minutes. Strain, cool, and serve. If you like, add a dash of honey.

Storage

Stored in a cool, dry place, Warm-Me-Up Herbal Tea should last for up to 1 year.

NOTE: *If you aren't a fan of the zing of ginger, replace up to half of it with peppermint for a milder taste.*

DIY Seed Bombs

Seed bombs are a fun, playful way to garden. Dried balls of clay and compost with seeds tucked inside, seed bombs can be tossed into the back corners of your garden or a long-forgotten flowerbed. After the seeds germinate, the bombs "explode" with colorful flowers and useful herbs growing in your garden.

SUPPLIES

- ❀ Clay
- ❀ Compost
- ❀ Old dishpan, storage tub, or mixing bowl
- ❀ Native, non-invasive flower or herb seeds (Try monarda, wild yarrow, or other indigenous species; or experiment with easy-to-grow garden medicinals, such as calendula, chamomile, or holy basil.)
- ❀ Watering can (optional)

> Make seed bombs in any quantity. Expect a yield of approximately 25 seed balls from 4 ounces of soil mix.

Instructions

We'll craft our seed bombs in three easy (but messy!) steps. Work outside or prepare your work area with a drop cloth or old tablecloth to simplify cleanup if things get a little wild.

Mix

1. Make your soil mix by combining 2 parts clay with 3 parts compost in an old bowl or bin. Be careful not to breathe in the clay dust, which can easily become airborne and irritate the lungs if poured too quickly.

2. Stir with your hands until the mixture is uniform.

3. Sprinkle with water until a damp, moldable consistency is formed. We're not making a mud puddle here, so take it slow! Shoot for the consistency of a very moist chocolate cake. It should hold together when squeezed in your hand.

Shape

There are two ways to add your seeds and form your balls. Method 1 is easier for young children, while Method 2 offers a little more control for older kids and adults.

Method 1:

1. Sprinkle your seeds across your soil medium and stir to combine, using approximately 50 to 75 seeds for every 4 ounces of soil mix.

2. To form balls, grab a small handful or a large pinch of the seeded soil medium, enough to make a 1-inch seed ball.

3. Firmly squeeze and roll the soil into a ball. Set aside to dry.

Method 2:

1. Gather a small handful or a large pinch of the soil medium in the palm of your hand, enough to make a 1-inch seed ball.

2. Sprinkle with 2 to 3 seeds and firmly squeeze and roll the soil mix into a ball, tucking the seeds inside. Set aside to dry.

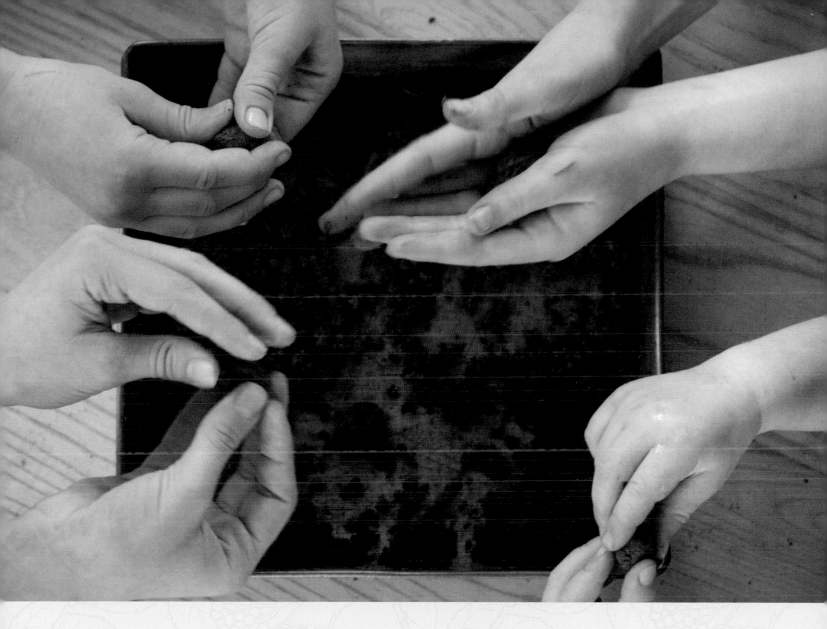

Dry

Let your seed balls aside to dry in a warm place for at least 24 hours before using. When thoroughly dry, seed balls can be placed in labeled waxed paper bags, tied with twine, and given as gifts!

Toss

To use your seed bombs, toss them into the corners of your yard or garden or other places you have permission to plant. Let the herbal revolution begin!

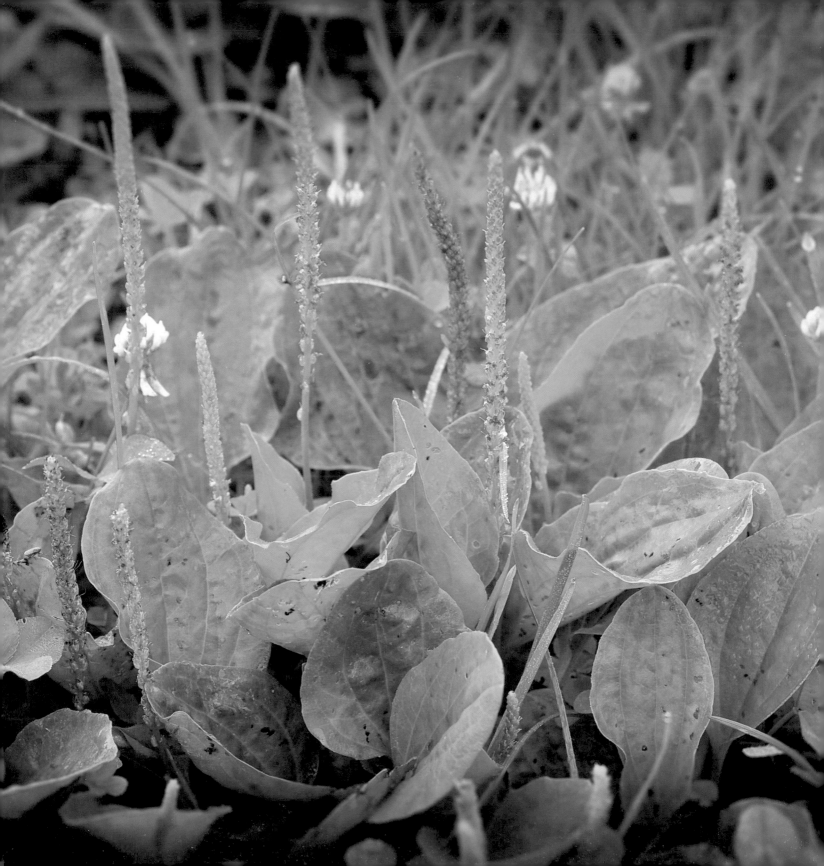

9 Plantain

Hello up there! It's me. Plantain. I'm right here, underneath your feet. You probably didn't even notice me. (That happens all the time!) But there's no need to apologize. I'm as tough as they come, and I don't mind being walked on now and then, as long as you also use me for more than a footpath.

Though I originally came from Europe, I have happily made my home from one side of North America to the other, hitching rides with European colonists as they moved westward hundreds of years ago. Anywhere these newcomers traveled I was sure to be found, since my seeds mixed in with their hay, garden seeds, and belongings, and then dropped out along the trail.

Even though I'm not from around here, I do try to make myself useful. I'm a handy plant to reach for when you need a remedy in a hurry. While I have as many uses as I do seeds, I'm simply the best for drawing out slivers, stingers, or infections. And since I'm so easy to find, you are almost guaranteed to stumble upon me when you need me the most.

I'm also edible (though perhaps not the most flavorful herb around), and a welcome plant for soothing tummies, earaches, and tickly coughs. Try adding my early spring leaves to your salads or my dried leaves to your tea blends. An infusion of my oil is a must for salves and creams.

Latin Name:

Plantago major

Parts Used:
leaves and seeds

Energetics:
cool and moist

Plantain leaf is a helpful herb for:
- Drawing out splinters and stingers
- Treating infections
- Soothing damaged skin
- Soothing the digestive tract
- Treating diarrhea
- Providing vitamins and minerals to the body
- Treating coughs

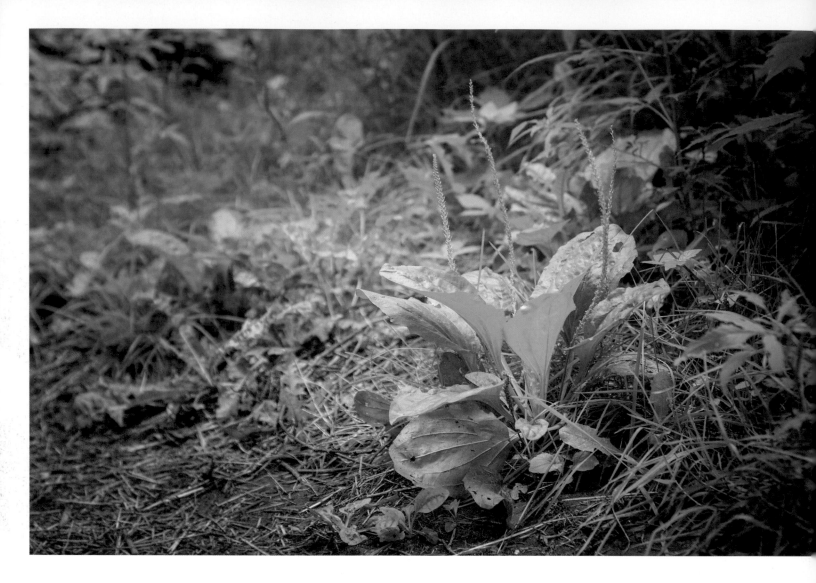

My Latin name is *Plantago major*. I think it's easy to remember because *Plantago* sounds a lot like "plantain," and *major* because I am a major help to have around! (My taller, thinner cousin, narrow leaf plantain, or *Plantago lanceolata*, is just as useful if I'm not close at hand.)

One easy way to be sure you've found me and not another plant is to remember my nickname, "frog's fiddle." If you slowly pull one of my leaves in half horizontally, you'll see some whit veins or threads connecting the two halves of my leaf. If they don't break, they look like strings on a fiddle for a cheerful frog to play!

I'll see you again soon. (I promise!)

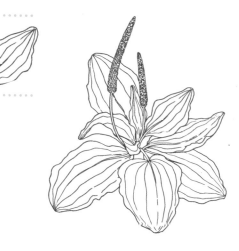

Field Identification

To identify plantain in the field, look for its key distinguishing characteristics. (Use the photograph below as a guide.)

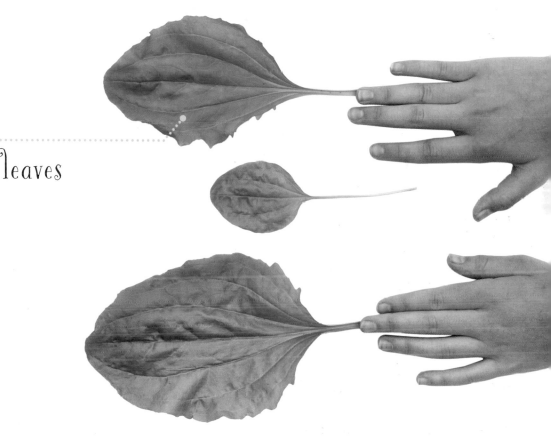

leaves

Leaves:

Plantain leaves are large, somewhat thick, and almond-shaped. The upper side of the leaf is smooth, with parallel veins. The underside of the leaf shows the veins more clearly as thick, raised, lighter-colored stripes. If you tear a leaf in half, these thick veins often protrude from one side of the leaf, like the strings on a stalk of celery. Plantain leaves are hairless.

Leaf stalk:

The thick veins in the plantain leaf continue down the leaf stalk, which turns red to pinkish toward the base. A cross-section is U-shaped, again reminiscent of a celery stalk.

Flower stalk:

A rough seed-covered spike emerges from the center of the rosette in summer, turning from green to tan as the season progresses.

Growth habit:

Leaves emerge from the ground in a basal rosette (or rose-shaped cluster of leaves). While the leaves have an elongated leaf stalk, the plant itself is stemless.

Habitat:

Plantain prefers poor, dry soil but can live in a variety of conditions. Plantain loves disturbed habitats, such as parks, lawns, trails, and roadways.

Range:

Plantain grows throughout North America and Europe.

Plantain Spit Poultice

Perhaps the simplest and most reached-for remedy in our household, plantain spit poultices come to the rescue again and again. When you're on the go and injuries happen, you don't always have a first aid kit on hand. But if you look around you'll likely find plantain! This is our go-to when we're surprised by a wasp sting, skinned knee, or sliver while adventuring away from home.

INGREDIENTS

- 1 or 2 fresh plantain leaves

TIME: Less than 1 minute, not including foraging time | **YIELD:** Approximately 1 teaspoon

Instructions

1. Pick a healthy, fresh plantain leaf. (Be sure you harvested your leaf from a place free of pets and lawn chemicals, and away from busy roads.)

2. Double-check that your plantain is free of debris and dirt. Rinse with fresh water if desired, and then pop it into your mouth.

3. Chew until the leaf becomes a thick green paste. It won't be your favorite flavor, but it's worth it—I promise!

4. Slather the paste onto bee stings, splinters, or other irritations. If desired, cover with a bandage. Reapply as needed.

Variation: The Spit-Free Spit Poultice

If the idea of putting on a remedy that has been chewed up and spit out is too much for you, don't fret. You can still benefit from a fresh herbal poultice, sans saliva. The method you use is entirely up to you! For the record, we think the first version is more fun, simple, and effective. (Unless, of course, you're squeamish!)

INGREDIENTS

- 1 or 2 fresh plantain leaves

Instructions

1. Pick a healthy, fresh plantain leaf. (Be sure you harvested your leaf from a place free of pets and lawn chemicals, and away from busy roads.)

2. Double-check that your plantain is free of debris and dirt, rinse with fresh water, and then coarsely chop with a kitchen knife.

3. Grind up the plantain with a mortar and pestle or food processor with a drop or two of water.

4. Apply as described above.

Plantain Wound Wash

Skinned knees, poison ivy, and other small injuries are no fun to clean! But removing dirt and debris is important to prevent infection and help you heal in a hurry. The next time you have a scrape or a rash, use this herbal wound wash to clean away dirt, speed healing, and help you feel better—fast.

TIME: Less than 30 minutes, not including foraging and drying time
YIELD: Approximately 1½ cups

Instructions

1. Place the plantain leaf in a small glass or stainless steel pot.

2. Cover with water and place over medium-high heat. Bring to a simmer.

3. Cover, remove from heat, and steep until warm to the touch, approximately 20 minutes.

4. Strain your warm infusion through a fine-mesh strainer, gently pressing your herbs to extract as much liquid as possible.

To use

Dip a clean, soft cloth into the infusion until saturated. Wring out slightly, and then gently drape over wounds, bee stings, or poison ivy. Always use a fresh cloth to prevent cross-contamination. Alternately, transfer the infusion to a wide bowl or basin and soak the affected area.

Repeat as desired to ease discomfort and speed healing.

Discard any leftover infusion, making a fresh batch for each application.

Flower and Leaf Paper Dolls

SUPPLIES

- Pressed or fresh flowers, leaves, seedpods, and other treasures
- Photocopies of Herbal Paper Dolls, found on page 137
- White glue or glue stick (optional)

This trio of paper dolls (designed just for you by artist Lucky Nielson) is ready to play! Dress them up with pressed leaves and flowers, tree branches, moss, or an acorn cap. Create flower bonnets and bloomers, herbal overalls and bunny ears, or leafy shoes and fairy wings.

Instructions

1. Make several photocopies of the Herbal Paper Dolls found at right. Leave your dolls together on the page, or cut to separate the individual dolls.

2. Dress them up with fresh or dried herbal decorations.

3. If desired, use white glue or a glue stick to permanently affix dried leaves and flowers.

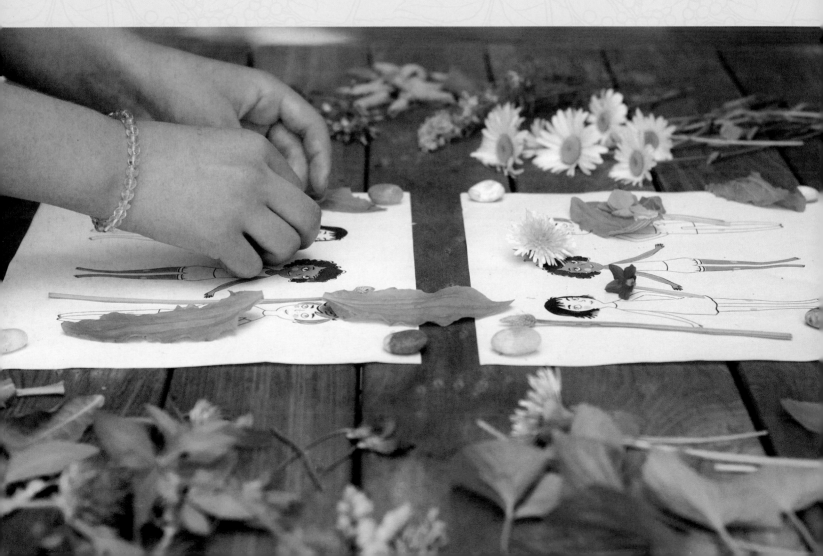

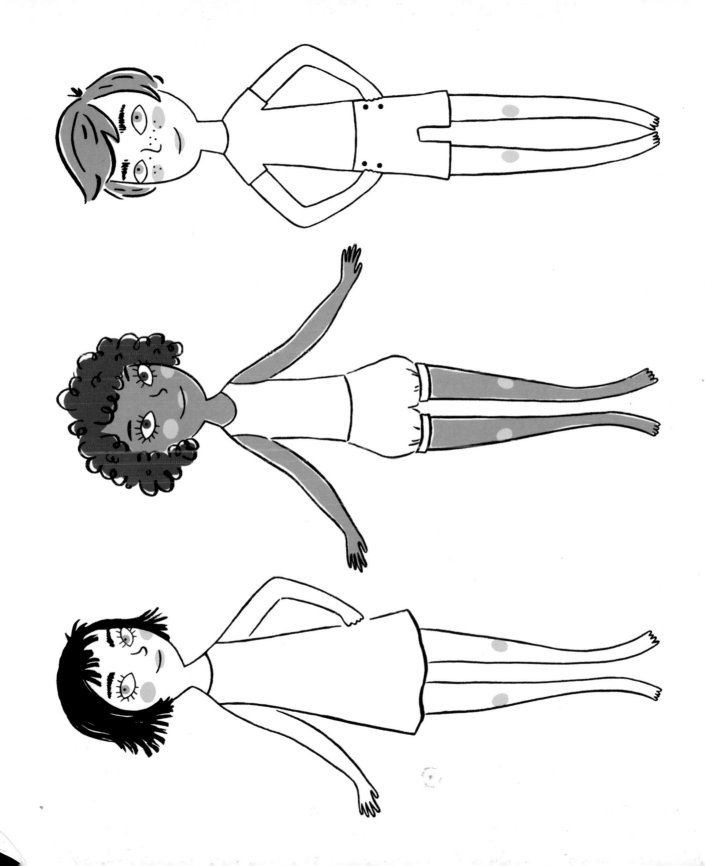

Splinter and Sting Salve

Slivers, stings, and bug bites are an unfortunate, but expected, part of life outdoors. Keep this homemade balm at the ready and the injuries won't be nearly as bad as you expected! The secret? Plantain leaf and activated charcoal. This dynamic duo helps pull splinters and stingers to the surface of the skin, while soothing irritation. Try it on minor skin infections too, such as picked scabs or ripped cuticles.

STEP 1: INFUSE YOUR OIL

ACTIVE TIME: Less than 1 hour, not including foraging and drying or wilting time
TOTAL TIME: 24 hours, or 3 to 4 weeks, depending on infusion method | **YIELD:** 5 ounces

INGREDIENTS

- ½ cup fresh, wilted, chopped plantain leaf, or scant ¼ cup dried
- 1 cup organic olive oil

Infused oils are among the easiest plant remedies to make. Using the ingredients listed below, follow the instructions on pages 169 or 170 to create yours. Choose whichever method you prefer: solar or stovetop.

STEP 2: MAKE YOUR BALMS

ACTIVE TIME: Less than 30 minutes | **TOTAL TIME:** 1 hour

INGREDIENTS

- ½ cup plantain-infused oil
- 1 tablespoon plus 1 teaspoon grated beeswax
- ½ teaspoon activated charcoal
- 8 drops peppermint essential oil (optional)
- 6 drops lavender essential oil (optional)

After your oil is infused and strained, it's time to create your balms!

1. Combine the plantain-infused oil and beeswax in a small, stainless steel or glass pan.

2. Warm over very low heat until the beeswax has melted.

3. Remove from heat.

4. Carefully measure the activated charcoal into the warmed oil and beeswax mixture. Whisk gently to combine. (Work slowly and carefully, as activated charcoal is profoundly messy when spilled!)

5. When the charcoal and oil are thoroughly combined, add the essential oils. Gently swirl or stir to combine.

6. Carefully pour the mixture into small glass jars or metal tins. If the balm hardens during pouring, simply rewarm over very low heat until melted.

7. Allow the balms to sit undisturbed until cool, and then lid and label.

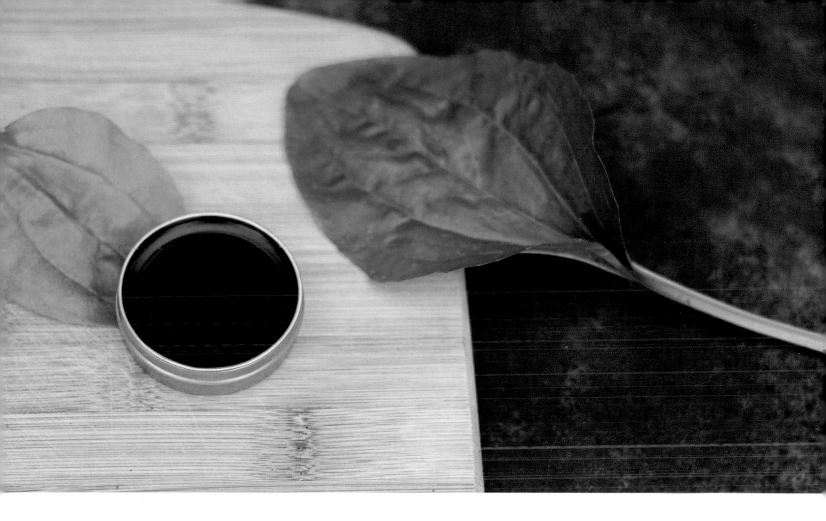

o use

...ply liberally as needed to splinters, bee
...ings, insect bites, or boils. Cover with a
...andage, as charcoal may stain clothing
... left exposed. Reapply as desired until
...scomfort is gone, or (for splinters) until
...e foreign body has emerged. Avoid the
...yes and eye area.

Storage

Stored in a cool, dry place, Splinter and
Sting Salve should last for up to 1 year.

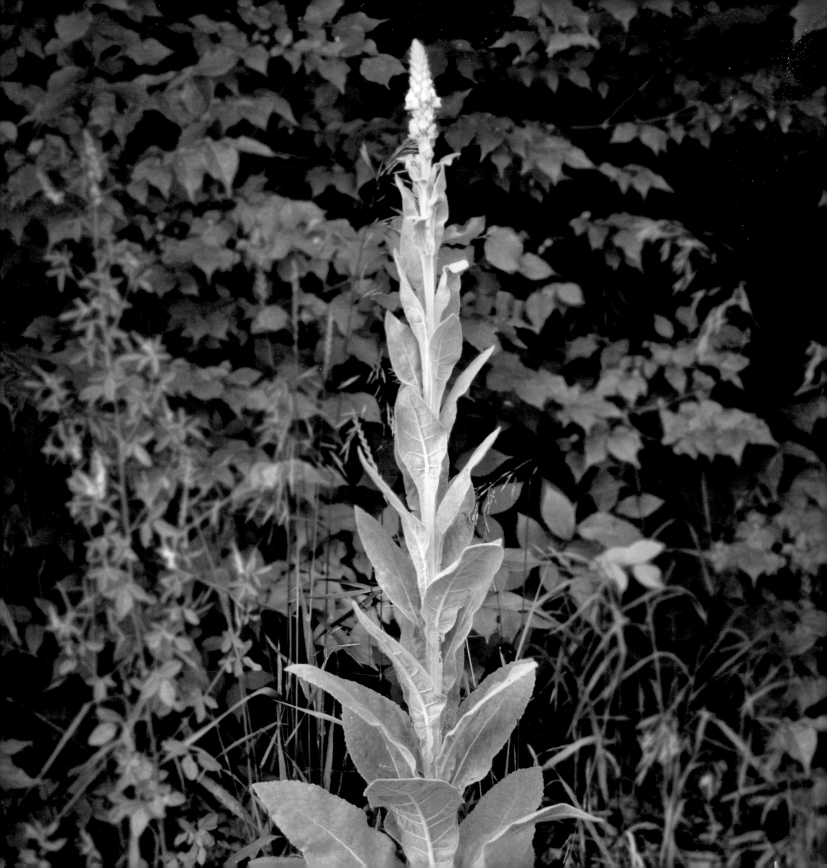

10 Mullein

Hello there! What brings you 'round these parts? I'm glad to see you, of course. It's just that I don't often have company in these sandy, dry places where I like to grow.

I see you're looking at my leaves. They're so fuzzy and soft—like a bouncesy flannel shirt. Go ahead and feel them! I don't mind a bit. In fact, if you'd like to take a few home, I'd be happy to share. Just be sure you leave enough for me to get by on. I am rather fond of them.

I have many nicknames, most on account of my fuzzy leaves. For obvious reasons, I'd prefer not to discuss "lumberjack's toilet paper." My less embarrassing nicknames include "flannel leaf," "poor man's blanket," and "Quaker's rouge." Rouge, or blush, is makeup used to make your cheeks

pink. Years back, folks used to rub my leaves on their cheeks to rosy them up.

But I can think of far finer uses for my leaves! Like making a tea for when you have a cough, for starters. My leaves may look simple, but they're one of the best cough remedies around. They're even used as a treatment for mild cases of asthma.

It's more than just my leaves that are helpful. Infused in oil, my flowers make the best earache remedy around. Because they don't all bloom at once, I suppose that means you'll have to come back to see me now and then. I'd like that!

Latin Name:

Verbascum thapsus

Parts Used:
leaves and flowers

Energetics:
cool and dry

Mullein is a helpful herb for:
- Treating coughs
- Comforting colds
- Soothing mild cases of asthma
- Reducing earaches

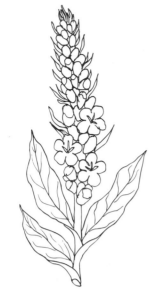

Field Identification

To identify mullein in the field, look for its key distinguishing characteristics. (Use the photographs on the right as a guide.)

Leaves:

Mullein leaves are large, elongated, and velvety. They are a soft, sage-green color and covered on both sides with a dense coating of soft hairs. When examining the underside of the leaves, you will find prominent veins that are raised and lighter in color than the rest of the leaf.

Stem:

Each second-year mullein plant produces a single stem that can grow over 6 feet tall. The stem is thick and brittle and bears velvety leaves. Leaves at the bottom are larger than those at the top. The upper 6 to 12 inches of the stem produces flowers.

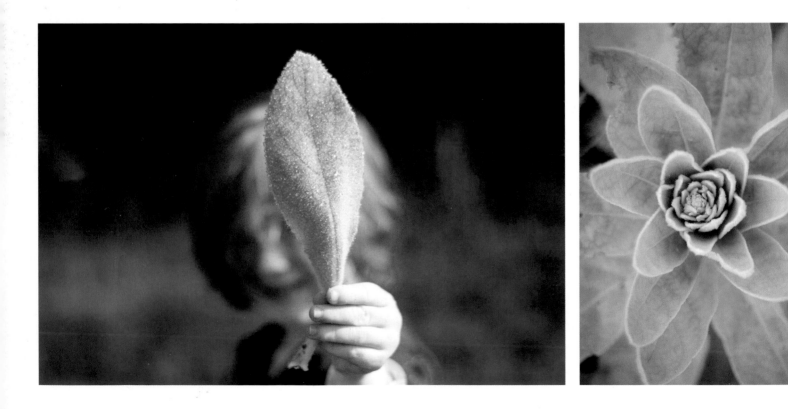

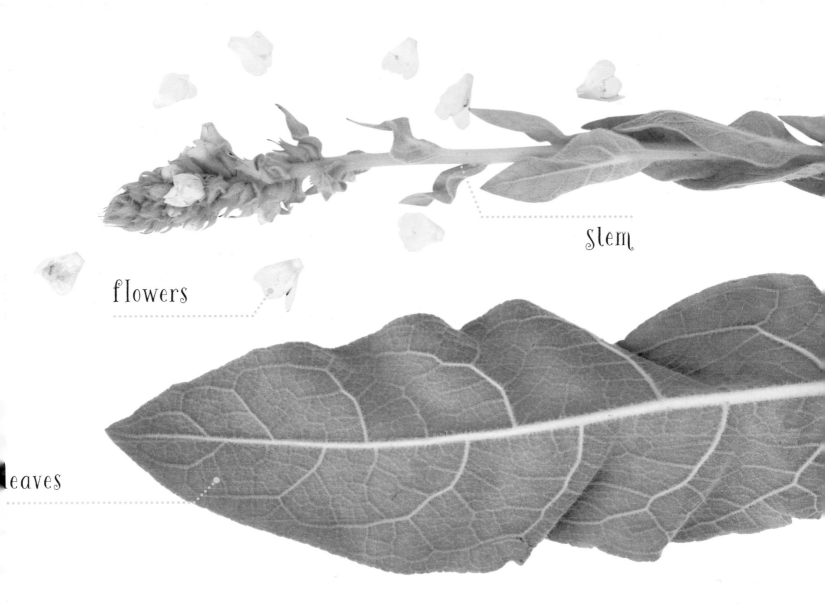

stem

flowers

leaves

Flowers:
Mullein flowers are five-petaled and yellow. Many are produced by a single flower stalk. The flowers do not all open at once, but instead open sporadically along the flower stalk.

Growth habit:
Mullein is a biennial (two-year) plant. During the first year, a basal rosette grows, formed of leaves only. On the second year, a flower stalk emerges from this rosette of leaves, bearing flowers and, later, seeds.

Habitat:
Mullein grows abundantly in full sun and dry, broken soil: along roadsides, ditches, and at the edges of fields.

Range:
Common mullein is found throughout much of the world, including most of North America.

Mullein Steam

When your nose and sinuses are congested and your cough won't quit, try a soothing mullein steam. Warm, moist, and comforting, a steam goes to the heart of the issue to clear out the gunk and help you breathe easy again.

INGREDIENTS

- ✤ 1 cup dried mullein leaf
- ✤ 2 tablespoons dried bee balm (optional)
- ✤ 2 tablespoons dried sage (optional)
- ✤ 1 gallon water

> Suitable for older children and adults only, due to the presence of hot liquid so close to face and hands.

ACTIVE TIME: Less than 10 minutes, not including foraging and drying time
TOTAL TIME: Less than 45 minutes | **YIELD:** Makes enough for one steam

Instructions

1. Combine all ingredients with the water in a large cooking pot. Be careful not to inhale the mullein dust, which can be irritating to the lungs.

2. Cover and bring to a boil over high heat.

3. Simmer for 3 to 4 minutes, and then remove from heat and allow to steep (covered) for an additional 5 minutes.

To use

Place a small, stable cooking pot on a folded towel or hot pad on a sturdy table. (Ensure that the bowl is level and stable before filling.) Transfer several cups of hot liquid into the bowl. (No need to strain.) Create a tent over your head using a large bath towel, and then carefully lower your face to a safe distance above the steaming bowl of water. Inhale the soothing steam.

Exercise caution, as you will be leaning over a pot of hot liquid, and burns are possible.

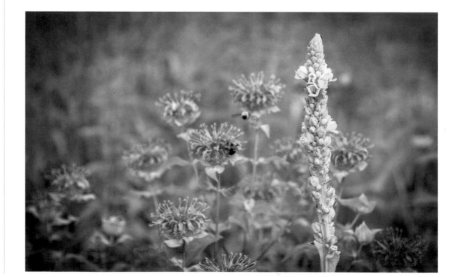

Chest Cold Tea

INGREDIENTS

- ¼ cup dried mullein leaf
- 2 tablespoons dried bee balm flower and leaf
- 1½ tablespoons licorice root
- 1 tablespoon cinnamon chips
- 1 tablespoon dried sage leaf

The herbs in this tea pack an immune-boosting punch and are also helpful for soothing achy chests and sore throats during bouts of cough and cold. While mullein, bee balm, and sage do the hard work of making you feel well, cinnamon and licorice root make each sip something to savor.

TIME: Less than 10 minutes, not including foraging and drying time
YIELD: Approximately ⅓ cup dry tea blend

Instructions

1. Measure all the ingredients into a clean, dry mixing bowl.
2. Crush any large leaves between your fingers if necessary and stir well to combine.
3. Transfer to a clean glass jar.
4. Lid and label.

To use

To brew, set a kettle of fresh water to boil. Measure 1 tablespoon of tea blend into a tea strainer or directly into a teapot. Pour 2 cups hot water over the tea, and then cover and steep for 10 minutes. Strain, cool, and serve. If you like, add a dash of honey.

Storage

Stored in a cool, dry place, Chest Cold Tea should last for up to 1 year.

Herbal Apothecary Jars

SUPPLIES

- ❋ Assortment of colorful dried herbs and flowers of your choice
- ❋ Small corked bottle or vial
- ❋ Craft glue
- ❋ Tweezers (optional)
- ❋ Small screw eye (optional)
- ❋ Hemp cord or yarn (optional)

A pretty, corked bottle or tiny glass jar is a lovely way to showcase beautiful sprigs or colorful layers of dried herbs. Let your imagination lead you! Line a few of your creations up along your dresser to remind you of your new herbal allies, or suspend one from a string and hang it in your window.

Instructions

1. Arrange an assortment of lovely dried herbs and tiny flowers on a plate or tray.

2. Using tweezers or your fingers, layer the herbs in the bottle as desired. Try creating an herbal rainbow, or feature just one or two of the species that you love most.

3. When you are satisfied with your arrangement, glue the cork into place and allow to dry.

4. If desired, twist a screw eye into the center of the cork and secure with craft glue. Hang your jar from a piece of hemp cord or yarn to display.

Variation

Instead of a tiny glass bottle containing an assortment of herbs, you can create a display of individual favorite herbs using larger bottles and decorative typed or handwritten tags.

Insert larger herbal specimens into bottles or jars, and then slip your herbal ID tag inside, or hang it from the neck of the bottle. Display on a shelf as a lovely reminder of your new herbal friends.

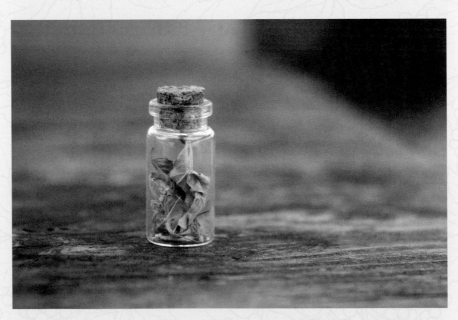

Mullein Leaf Cough Syrup

This easy-to-make cough syrup is a gentle, but effective, way to clear and comfort an icky, wet cough. And because it's made with flavorful herbs and throat-soothing honey, it tastes fantastic too. As one young friend said, "I wish all cough syrup tasted this good!"

TIME: Less than 30 minutes, not including foraging and drying time
YIELD: Approximately 2¼ cups

INGREDIENTS

- ¼ cup dried mullein leaf
- ¼ cup wild cherry bark
- ¼ cup white pine needles and bark (optional, but recommended)
- 3 tablespoons licorice root
- 2 tablespoons sage leaf
- 1 tablespoon thyme
- 3 cups water
- ¾ to 1 cup raw honey

Instructions

1. Combine all ingredients except the honey in a nonreactive saucepan and bring to a simmer.

2. Simmer uncovered until the water has reduced to roughly half of its original amount, or 1¼ cups, approximately 15 to 20 minutes.

3. Cool slightly, and then strain out the herbs through a fine-mesh strainer lined with a thin cotton cloth. Squeeze to extract as much liquid as possible and compost or discard the solids.

4. Measure your liquid. You should have approximately 1½ cups. Add additional water, if needed, to bring the liquid volume back up to 1½ cups.

5. When the decoction is just warm to the touch, add ¼ cup of honey for every ½ cup of decoction. (Example: If your yield was 1½ cups, add ¾ cup of honey. If your yield was 2 cups, add 1 cup of honey.)

6. Stir to combine. Transfer to a clean glass jar, lid, and label.

Talk to your midwife or doctor before using during pregnancy.

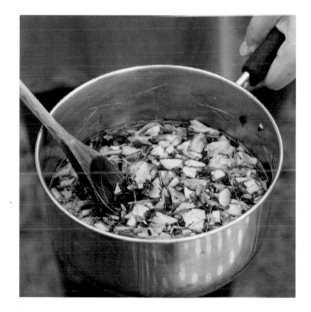

To use

Adults take 2 teaspoons each hour as needed. Children over two years of age take 1 teaspoon each hour as needed. Because this formula contains honey, it is not appropriate for children under one year of age.

Storage

Store in the refrigerator for up to 3 months. Freeze for up to 1 year.

Mullein-Garlic Ear Oil

If you've ever had an earache you know you want relief in a hurry! The dull ache or stabbing pain is difficult to endure. But don't despair. This herb-and-garlic oil reduces pain and inflammation fast. It's one remedy that my family never wants to be without.

ACTIVE TIME: Less than 20 minutes, not including foraging and drying time
TOTAL TIME: 35 minutes to overnight | **YIELD:** ½ cup

INGREDIENTS

- 3 medium cloves of garlic
- 2 teaspoons dried or fresh mullein flowers
- ½ cup olive oil

Instructions

1. Peel and mince the garlic and allow to rest for 15 minutes.

2. Combine all the ingredients in a small saucepan. Gently warm over a double boiler or very low heat until warm, but not hot, to the touch. Be careful not to overheat!

3. Turn off heat, cover, and infuse overnight. If you need your oil sooner, allow to steep covered for a minimum of 15 minutes.

4. Strain your oil carefully and transfer to a clean glass jar or bottle, and label.

Not for use with a punctured eardrum. Not appropriate for treating swimmer's ear (a bacterial ear infection). To treat swimmer's ear, make a 1:1 combination of rubbing alcohol and white vinegar and drop into ears. Always treat both ears.

To use

Warm your jar or bottle of ear oil in a bowl of hot water. Test the temperature on the inside of your wrist. When it is comfortably warm—but not too hot—place four drops of warm ear oil in each ear. (Always treat both ears, as infections are easily transferred from one side to the other.) Gently massage outer ear and earlobe to help the oil work its way inside. Place a cotton ball in the outer ear to keep from dripping oil onto clothing or furniture. If using at bedtime, protect your pillow with an absorbent towel.

Storage

Store in the refrigerator for up to 1 year.

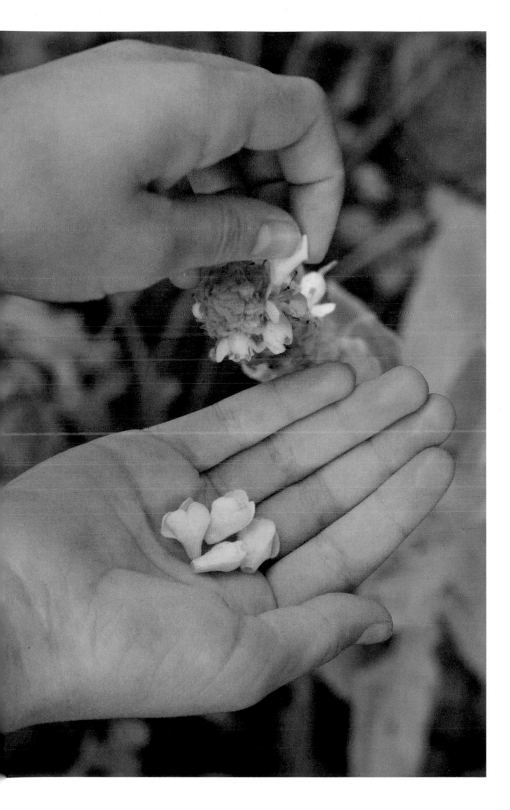

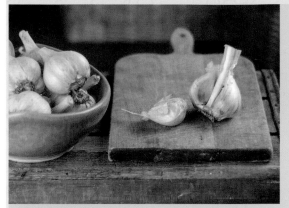

The Right Way to Prep Garlic

Garlic is famous for its immune-boosting powers and its antimicrobial and antibacterial qualities. But did you know that unless you prepare garlic properly, those benefits are lost? Most of us have been doing it wrong our whole lives.

To activate garlic's superpowers, slice, chop, or crush the fresh cloves and allow the garlic to sit for 15 minutes to activate the allicin, garlic's powerful enzyme.

Heating garlic immediately after chopping means you lose out on the biggest health benefits of this wonderful herb!

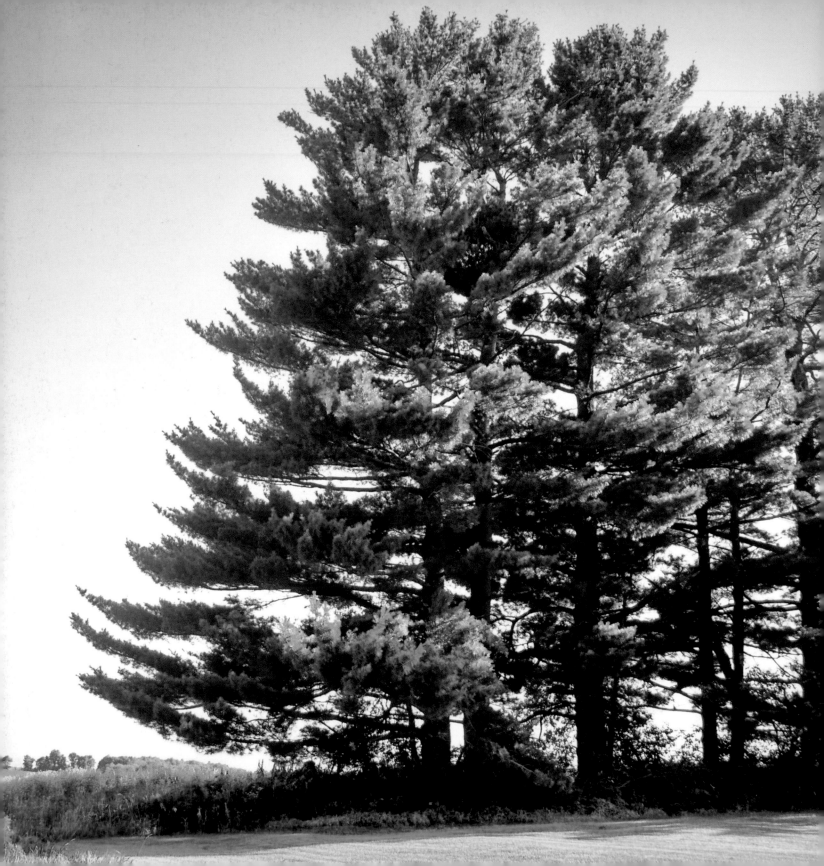

11 White Pine

Hello, old friend. I am Strobus, the eastern white pine, tall and proud and strong. My roots are deep, and even in the fiercest storms I am both steadfast and yielding. I have lived on this land since time began and have stood guard over many generations.

I am but one of a family of more than one hundred pine species, growing throughout most of the world. Beyond my family of pines, I have many conifer cousins, also bearing needles and cones: hemlock, spruce, fir, tamarack, and cedar. These are not pines, but "evergreens," as you call them, of other families.

To tell pine apart from our conifer cousins, you need only look at our needles. Only those with needles grown in bundles (or "fascicles") are truly pine.

My needles, like the letters of my common name, come in fives. Five needles per fascicle, five letters in the word "white." W-H-I-T-E. If you touch my needles, you will find they are soft and gentle, much like my medicine.

Reach for me when your lungs are weary—during times of cough and cold. With my abundance of vitamin C, I am a tonic when you are weakened by cold, cough, or flu. I will bring you the strength of the white pine when you need it most.

Latin Name:

Pinus strobus

Parts Used:
needles, bark, and resin

Energetics:
warm and dry

Pine is a helpful herb for:
- Soothing aching lungs
- Calming coughs
- Nourishing the body with vitamin C (five times the concentration of lemons!)
- Supplying the body with vitamin A

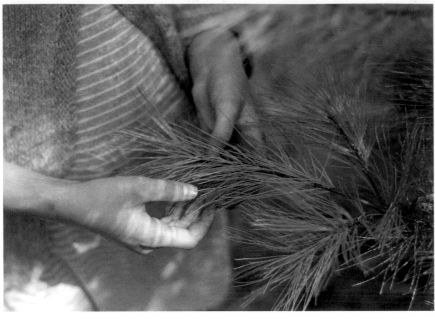
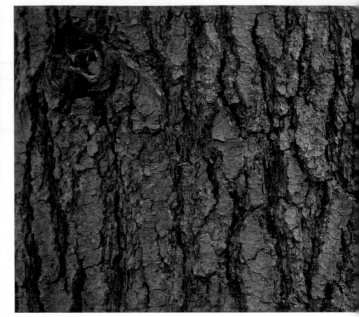

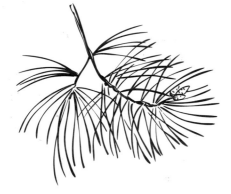

Field Identification

To identify white pine in the field, look for its key distinguishing characteristics. (Use the photographs above as a guide.)

Bark and trunk:
The bark of a young white pine is smooth and greenish-gray. A mature tree bears rough gray-brown to reddish-brown bark that is deeply grooved by irregular vertical cracks.

Needles:
Eastern white pine needles are soft to the touch and grow in fascicles of five. Each needle is 3 to 5 inches long, flexible, and thin.

Scent:
The scent of white pine is woodsy and warm. Not as strong as cedar, it is still a delightful evergreen scent.

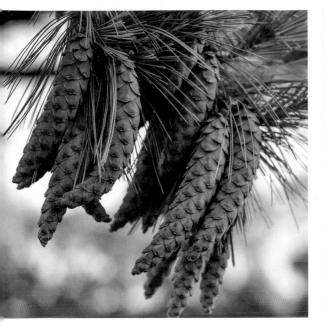

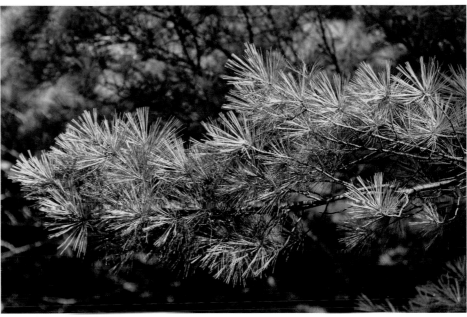

Cones:

Cones are elongated and tapered, to 6 inches in length. They are green when young and ripen to tan when mature. White pine cones lack the sharp prickles that are on each scale of other species.

Growth habit:

Eastern white pine grows 50 to 80 feet tall. Unlike the classic "Christmas tree" shape of many other conifers, white pines have a broader, more rounded crown.

Habitat:

White pine grows in well-drained, slightly acidic soil. You will find the trees growing on ridges, in forests, and in most towns or cities.

Range:

White pine is native to the eastern half of North America, but can be found planted in other regions as well. If you do not live in a region where white pine grows, substitute any available pine species in the recipes that follow. (Yew, however, is toxic. This evergreen shrub produces small red berries and short, wide, dark needles arranged along each branch.)

Lookalikes:

To a beginner at tree identification, white pine resembles many other conifer species. A close inspection of the needles is your best identifier. Are the needles growing in fascicles? Then it is a pine. How many needles per fascicle? If it's five (and you're in the United States east of the Mississippi River), it is probably white pine.

Substitutions:

No white pine in your neighborhood? No problem! Any of the true pine species can be substituted for white pine in the recipes that follow.

Woodland Soak and Steam

INGREDIENTS

- 🌿 1 cup chopped fresh or dried pine needles and small branches
- 🌿 1 cup juniper or spruce branches and berries (optional)
- 🌿 3 tablespoons dried bee balm (optional)
- 🌿 2 tablespoons dried thyme
- 🌿 1 gallon water

When your nose is stuffy and your head is congested, a warm steam or bath can make all the difference! This forest-scented steam will help you breathe easy—and feel better soon. This steam bath is suitable for adults and older children only, due to the presence of such hot liquids so close to faces and hands. For younger children, follow the method below for the Woodland Soak.

ACTIVE TIME: Less than 10 minutes, not including foraging time
TOTAL TIME: 45 minutes | **YIELD:** Makes enough for one steam or bath

Instructions

1. Combine all ingredients with the water in a large cooking pot.

2. Bring to a boil over high heat.

3. Reduce heat to low and simmer for 15 minutes, covered.

4. Remove from heat and allow to steep (covered) for an additional 20 minutes.

To use

For Woodland Soak
Fill the bathtub. Pour the infusion through a strainer and add liquids to bath water. Stir and adjust the temperature as needed. Now it's bath time!

For Woodland Steam
For older children and adults, inhaling herbal steam can be a comfort during times of congestion and sinus pressure. Exercise caution, as you will be leaning over a pot of hot liquid and burns are possible.

Place a heatproof bowl on a folded towel or hot pad on the table. Ensure that the bowl is stable before filling. Transfer several cups of hot liquid into the bowl. No need to strain. Create a tent over your head using a large bath towel, and then carefully lower your face to a safe distance above the steaming bowl of water. Inhale the soothing woodland steam.

Storage

Woodland Soak and Steam is best used immediately and made fresh as needed. However you may harvest and dry the herbs in advance. Ensure they are thoroughly dried, and then store in a lidded glass jar for up to 6 months in a cool, dry place.

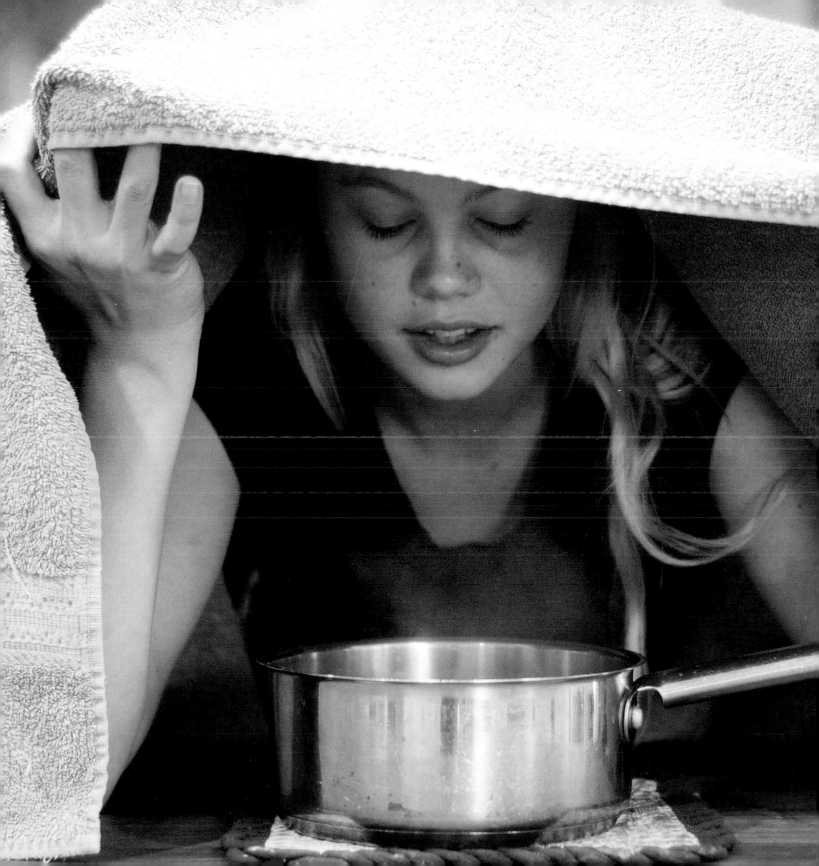

Nature's Paintbrushes

SUPPLIES

- Clipboard or large piece of cardboard and additional rubber bands
- Grasses, flowers, and leaves of your choice
- Craft scissors, branch cutter, or pocketknife
- Rubber bands, yarn, twine, or string
- Tempera or acrylic paints
- An old, heavy plate to use as a paint palette
- Paper

Is a paintbrush only something that we buy, or could a paintbrush be something more? Make your own from garden finds, such as seedpods, tree branches, leaves, and flowers. Or visit your local flower shop and ask if they have any spent flowers, ferns, or other trimmings to donate to your project. The only limit is your imagination!

Instructions

Set up your painting area.

Painting outdoors is a treat! Find a shady nook in which to set up your makeshift art studio. Attach your paper to a clipboard to keep it from blowing away, or improvise with a couple of large rubber bands and a sturdy piece of cardboard. If you prefer, work indoors on a protected surface.

Gather your natural materials.

Harvest some tree branches approximately the diameter of a drinking straw or slightly thinner. These will serve as your paintbrush handles. Choose species that don't exude sticky sap, and cut them neatly to the length you desire, using a knife or branch cutter.

Head into the garden with an eye for texture. Look for sturdy plants that will make for interesting textures when dipped into paint. The possibilities are endless!

Bristle materials can include:

- Grasses
- Leaves
- Pine needles
- Flowers
- Horsetails
- Ferns

Make your brushes and stamps.

To create your paintbrushes, use rubber bands, yarn, or twine to attach the bristles. Hold a cluster of leaves, needles, or other material at one end of the stick, and then tightly wrap and secure with yarn or a rubber band. Trim the end of the bristle if desired. Because there is no right or wrong way to make a paintbrush, you can assemble your own with little to no help from an adult.

Paint!

Choose two or three colors of paint and place a dime-sized dollop of each on your palette. Twist or dip your new brush into the paint and dab, swipe, and swirl away! Some results will be more pleasing than others, so keep experimenting. Natural paintbrushes don't offer the same control that we have come to expect from purchased brushes. The results tend to be abstract and a bit wild. As long as you're having fun, there is no wrong way to do it.

As each painting is completed it can be hung to dry on a sheltered clothesline or brought inside to dry to prevent it from blowing away in a breeze.

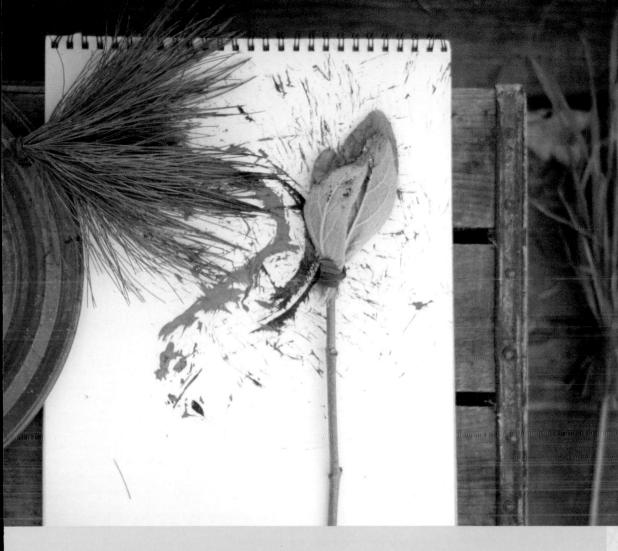

Variation: Natural Stamps

Making natural stamps is a simple but rewarding craft as well, and better suited for younger hands. Use larger, sturdy seedpods or fruits to create your own stamps.

To use, simply spread a small amount of paint on an old plate, dip your stamps, and print.

Suggestions for natural stamps include:

- Apples, crabapples, or pears, cut along the "equator" to reveal the star inside

- Sliced whole celery head for rose-like prints, or individual stalks for little moons

- Pine cones

- Flower seedpods (poppies are especially nice)

Woodland Vinegar

Vinegar is an important ingredient in countless kitchen recipes, adding acidity, improving texture, and boosting nutrition. From salad dressings and sauces to marinades for veggies and meat, vinegar is vital! This pine-infused vinegar tastes woodsy and delightful. Just a splash will add a delicious wild food flair (and lots of vitamin C) to your home-cooked meals.

ACTIVE TIME: Less than 10 minutes, not including foraging time
TOTAL TIME: 6 weeks | **YIELD:** 2 scant cups

INGREDIENTS

- ❧ 2 cups pine needles and fine branches, coarsely chopped to allow them to fit in your bottle or jar
- ❧ 2 cups raw apple cider vinegar (labeled "unpasteurized" or "with the mother")

Instructions

1. Pack pine needles and small branches tightly into a pint-sized jar and cover with vinegar.

2. Push any wayward needles under the surface of the vinegar and cover with a plastic lid or line a metal lid with a piece of a waxed paper, parchment, or a small plastic bag.

3. If your pine needles float, weigh them down with a clean, dry stone or smaller glass jar placed inside your pint jar.

4. Place in a cool dark place to infuse for 6 weeks, removing the weight and shaking occasionally.

5. After 6 weeks, strain your infused vinegar.

6. Compost or discard the solids and transfer the vinegar to a clean glass jar. Lid and label.

To use

Use as you would balsamic vinegar—for herbal salad dressings, marinades, or sauces. Or drizzle on sautéed vegetables.

Storage

Stored in a cool, dry place, Woodland Vinegar will keep for at least 1 year.

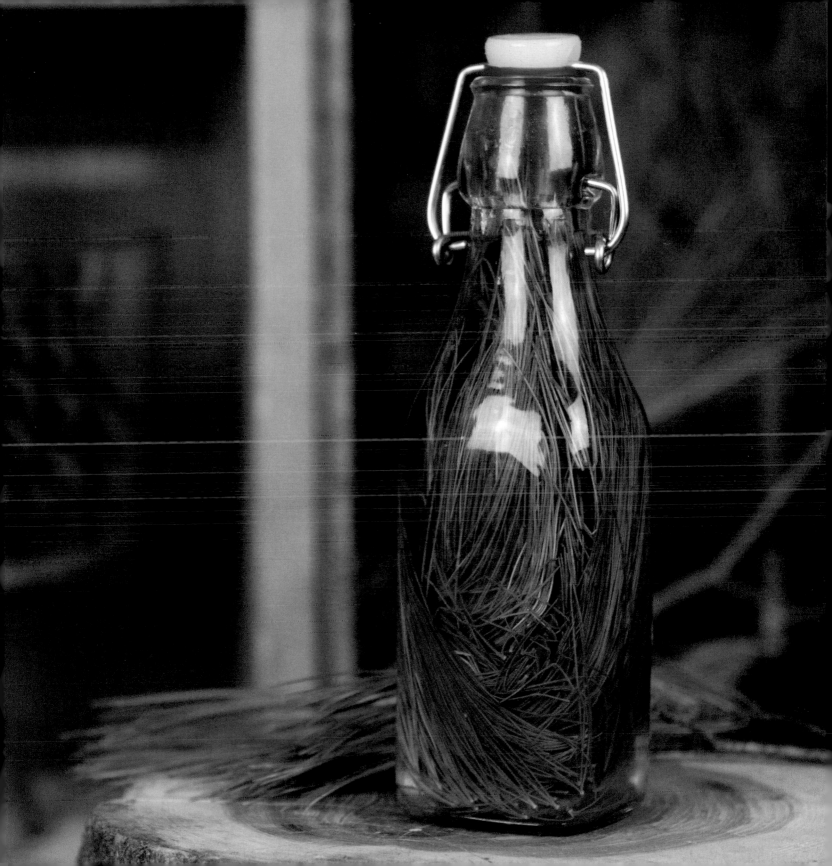

Pine Needle Tea

INGREDIENTS

- A handful of fresh white pine needles, still on the branch, approximately ¼ cup, chopped
- Approximately 3 cups of water

When my children and I take a walk in a pine forest, we inevitably come home with our pockets filled with fresh needles and twigs. Back home, we simmer up one of our favorite drinks: pine needle tea. This warm and woodsy drink is tasty with or without honey, and tastes like something a forest elf might enjoy. It's earthy, fragrant, and delicious! And since it's packed with vitamin, C, we drink it every time we have a cold.

TIME: Less than 10 minutes, not including foraging time
YIELD: Makes 2 generous mugs of tea

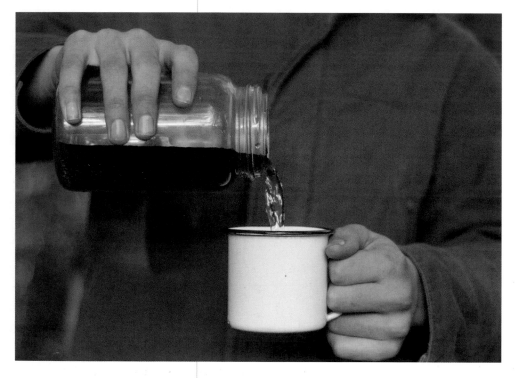

Instructions

1. Place the pine needles and small branches in a small saucepan.
2. Cover with the water.
3. Set over high heat and bring to a vigorous boil.
4. Reduce to a simmer, cover, and simmer gently for 5 minutes.
5. Remove from heat and allow to steep, covered for an additional 10 minutes.
6. Strain and serve warm, adding a touch of honey if desired. (Remember, no honey for children under one year of age.)

To use

Enjoy anytime, especially during cold and flu season, as a tasty way to get your vitamin C!

Citrus and Pine Shrub

Have you already tried the Sunshine Shrub? (If not, see page 88 to learn all about shrubs!) This shrub is that recipe's cousin: sweet, sour, and so refreshing. It's one of my family's favorite ways to rehydrate after exercise or on hot summer days. Like all shrubs, this recipe is made of fruit, vinegar, and a sweetener (raw honey). Add a splash to fizzy water and enjoy.

ACTIVE TIME: Less than 15 minutes, not including foraging time
TOTAL TIME: 10 days | **YIELD:** Approximately 3 cups

Instructions

1. Without removing the peels, coarsely chop the orange and lemon.

2. Place the citrus in a glass quart jar and muddle with the back of a wooden spoon, pressing gently to release some of the juices.

3. Pound the optional lemongrass stalk with the back of the knife and coarsely chop and add to the jar or add coriander seeds.

4. Add the pine, vinegar, and honey. Stir to dissolve the honey.

5. Cover with a plastic lid or line a metal lid with parchment, waxed paper, or a plastic bag, and place in the refrigerator for 10 days, shaking or stirring daily.

6. After the infusing period is complete, strain your shrub through a fine-mesh strainer, firmly pressing to extract as much juice as possible. Transfer to a clean, dry glass bottle or jar. Lid and label.

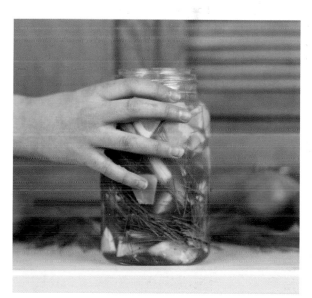

To use

Add 1 tablespoon shrub syrup to a cup of chilled, carbonated water and drink.

Storage

Stored in the refrigerator, homemade shrubs will keep for up to 6 months.

INGREDIENTS

- 1 large orange
- 1 Meyer lemon, or ½ regular lemon
- 1 lemongrass stalk or 2 teaspoons whole coriander (optional)
- ⅓ cup chopped fresh white pine needles and small twigs
- 1½ cups raw apple cider vinegar
- ¾ cup honey

Use with caution if any of the following conditions apply:

- Pregnancy
- Kidney stones
- Gallbladder issues
- Acid reflux
- Ulcers

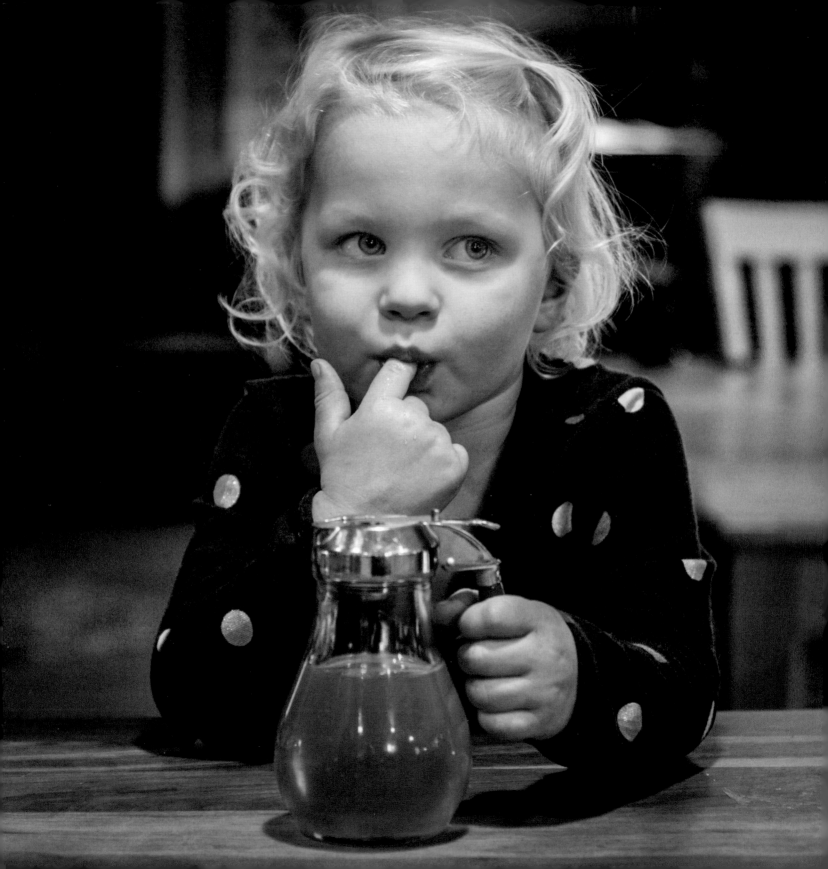

12 Basic Recipes

The recipes that follow can be made in any quantity, depending on the amount of herbs you have on hand and how much finished product you desire. From ¼ pint to ½ gallon or more, how much you make is up to you! To increase or decrease batch size, simply multiply or divide ingredients, while maintaining the same proportions.

A few warnings:

1. For the sake of safety, only experiment with herbs that you know are safe and healthy to ingest or apply to the skin, and plants that were harvested in an area free of chemical sprays, nearby traffic, and pet waste. And remember: not all parts of a useful plant are safe to ingest. Research herbs thoroughly before harvesting them for remedies or recipes.

2. A word about dosage: The appropriate amount to take of a remedy varies by age, weight, and constitution. Always start slowly when working with new herbs. When using plants not outlined in the previous chapters, consult with several herbal books that address the plant you are using to determine proper dosage. (See Resources, page 171, for book suggestions.)

3. If a remedy develops mold or an "off" smell at any stage of the process, discard and begin again.

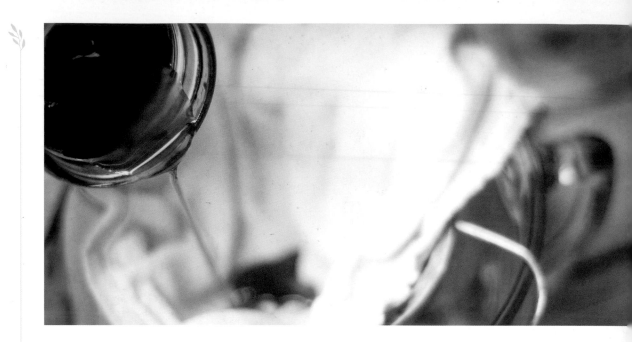

BASIC SYRUP: DECOCTION METHOD

A syrup is a soothing way to take more bitter herbs, or to take herbs designed to soothe the throat or quiet a cough. Decoction extraction is helpful for coaxing the beneficial compounds out of sturdy plant parts, such as roots, stems, and bark, and is useful for working with dried plant materials.

INGREDIENTS

- ½ cup fresh or dried leaf, root, flower, or berry of choice
- 3 cups water
- 1½ cups raw honey

TIME: Less than 30 minutes, not including foraging and wilting or drying time
YIELD: Approximately 3 cups

Instructions

1. Combine the herbs and water in a nonreactive saucepan.

2. Bring to a boil, and then reduce to a simmer.

3. Simmer until the volume of liquid has reduced by half.

4. Strain through a fine-mesh colander, pressing to extract as much liquid as possible from the herbs.

5. Cool until just warm (but not hot) and mix with honey.

6. Lid, label, and store in the refrigerator for up to 1 year.

Dosage

Dosage will vary by age and the plant type: 1 tablespoon for adults or 1 teaspoon for childre as needed, is a common dose. Contains honey. Not suitable for children under one year of age.

BASIC SYRUP: HONEY EXTRACTION METHOD

Syrups are helpful for quieting coughs, soothing sore throats, and making bitter or unpleasant herbs more tasty. This version is the simplest to make, using just fresh herbs and raw honey.

ACTIVE TIME: Less than 20 minutes, not including foraging and wilting time
TOTAL TIME: 4 weeks | **YIELD:** Approximately 1½ cups

INGREDIENTS

- 1½ cups fresh root, leaf, flower, or berry of choice
- 1½ to 2 cups raw honey, or enough to cover herbs

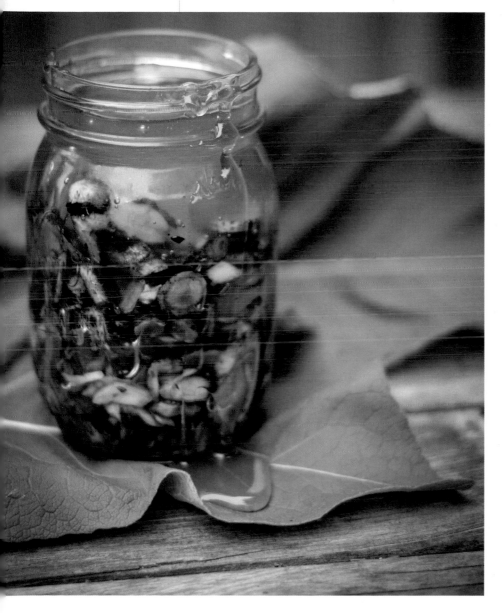

Instructions

1. Place the herbs in clean, dry mason jar. (Fill the jar only half to two-thirds full.)

2. Pour the raw honey into the jar, lid, and label.

3. Set on a counter out of direct sun and flip the jar over to mix once daily (or anytime you think of it) for 4 to 6 weeks.

4. Strain your honey, squeezing as much liquid goodness as you can out of the herbs. Compost or discard the solids.

5. Store on the counter for low-moisture herbs, or in the refrigerator for higher-moisture herbs (including roots, tubers, or bulbs) for up to 1 year.

Dosage

Dosage will vary by age and the plant type: 1 tablespoon for adults or 1 teaspoon for children, as needed, is a common dose. Contains honey. Not suitable for children under one year of age.

BASIC GLYCERITE: FRESH HERB METHOD

Glycerites are sweet, mild herbal remedies especially appropriate for kids. Made by infusing herbs in sweet glycerin syrup, they can be taken by the spoonful or stirred into applesauce or tea. This formula is for working with fresh herbs. See page 167 for instructions on making glycerites from dried herbs.

ACTIVE TIME: Less than 10 minutes, not including foraging and wilting time
TOTAL TIME: 6 weeks | **YIELD:** ¾ cup

INGREDIENTS

- 1½ cups fresh root, leaf, flower, or berry of choice
- 1 cup vegetable glycerin, or enough to cover herbs or berries

Instructions

1. Harvest herbs in the late morning, after the dew has dried. Shake off any dirt or debris, and then lay plants out on a cookie sheet to wilt in the shade for 12 to 24 hours.

2. After wilting, coarsely chop the plant material and place in a clean, dry glass jar, filling approximately two-thirds full.

3. Pour glycerin over the herbs, being sure to fully submerge all the leaves. Use a chopstick or butter knife to release any air bubbles.

4. Cover with a plastic lid or line a metal lid with a piece parchment, waxed paper, or plastic. Label the jar with the plant name and date, and place in an out-of-the-way corner of the kitchen.

5. Shake the jar daily (or as often as you think of it) for 6 weeks.

6. After 6 weeks, strain the glycerite through a cheesecloth-lined colander, squeezing as much liquid out of the herbs as you can. Compost or discard the herbs and transfer the glycerite to a clean glass jar or dropper bottles.

7. Lid and label.

To use

Glycerites may be taken straight or added to a cup of tea. They are also delicious stirred into applesauce.

Dosage

Dosage will vary by age and the plant type: 1 to 2 drops per 10 pounds of body weight for children is a common dose, taken up to 3 times per day, as needed. A common dose for adults is ½ teaspoon up to 5 times per day, as needed.

Storage

Stored in a cool, dry place, glycerites will keep for at least 1 year.

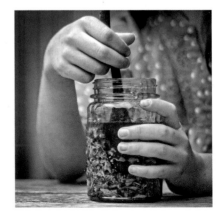

BASIC GLYCERITE: DRIED HERB METHOD

No fresh herbs? No problem! Glycerites are just as easy to make from dried herbs as they are from fresh. Adding water to the glycerin before pouring it over the herbs ensures that the herbs properly infuse.

ACTIVE TIME: Less than 10 minutes, not including foraging and drying time
TOTAL TIME: 6 weeks | **YIELD:** ¾ cup

INGREDIENTS

- ½ cup dried leaf, root, flower, or berry of your choice
- ¾ cup vegetable glycerin
- ¼ cup water

Instructions

1. Place the dried herbs in a clean, dry glass jar.

2. Combine glycerin and room-temperature water in a measuring pitcher and stir well to combine.

3. Pour the glycerin/water mixture over the dried herbs, being sure to fully submerge all the plants. Use a chopstick or butter knife to release any air bubbles.

4. Cover the jar with a tightly fitting lid and label with remedy type and date. Place in an out-of-the-way corner of the kitchen.

5. Shake the jar daily (or as often as you think of it) for 6 weeks.

6. After 6 weeks, strain the glycerite through a cheesecloth-lined colander, squeezing as much liquid out of the herbs as you can. Compost or discard the herbs and transfer the glycerite to a clean glass jar or dropper bottles.

7. Lid and label.

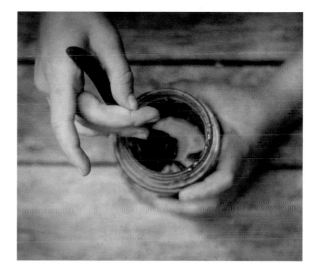

To use

Glycerites may be taken straight or added to a cup of tea. They are also delicious stirred into applesauce.

Dosage

Dosage will vary by age and the plant type: 1 to 2 drops per 10 pounds of body weight for children is a common dose, taken up to 3 times per day, as needed. A common dose for adults is ½ teaspoon up to 5 times per day, as needed.

Storage

Stored in a cool, dry place, glycerites will keep for at least 1 year.

BASIC OXYMEL

An oxymel is a plant extraction made with equal parts apple cider vinegar and honey. Vinegar is an excellent medium for extracting minerals from mineral-rich herbs. Also, the word "oxymel" is sure to impress your friends!

INGREDIENTS

- 2 cups fresh leaf, root, flower, or berry of choice or 1 cup dried
- 1 cup raw apple cider vinegar
- ½ cup raw honey

ACTIVE TIME: less than 10 minutes, not including foraging and wilting or drying time
TOTAL TIME: 4 to 6 weeks | **YIELD:** 1¼ cups

Instructions

1. Fill a glass jar two-thirds full with wilted or dried plant material.
2. Cover with vinegar and raw honey.
3. Cover with a plastic lid or line a metal lid with a piece of parchment, waxed paper, or plastic. Label the jar with the plant name and date.
4. Shake daily (or as often as you think of it) for 6 weeks to 6 months.
5. Strain the oxymel, squeezing as much liquid goodness as you can out of the herbs.
6. Taste your oxymel and add additional honey i desired, stirring to dissolve.
7. Discard the herbs and transfer the remedy to a clean glass jar and label.

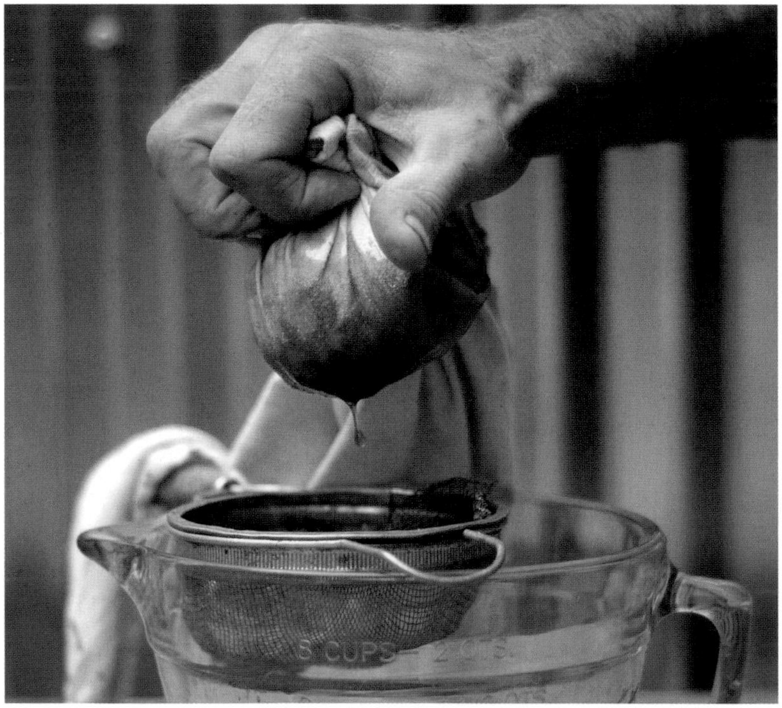

Storage

Stored in a cool, dry place, oxymels will keep indefinitely.

To use

Oxymels can be taken straight or stirred into water, tea, or juice.

Dosage

Dosage will vary by age and the plant type: 1 tablespoon as needed for adults or 1 teaspoon for children is a common dose. Contains honey. Not suitable for children under one year of age.

BASIC SOLAR-INFUSED OIL

Solar-infused oils may take a while, but the results are worth it! Try to start them as the plants reach their peak throughout the season, if you can. Solar-infused oils can also be made with dried herbs with good results, as long as the herbs are very fresh.

ACTIVE TIME: less than 10 minutes, not including foraging and wilting or drying time
TOTAL TIME: 3 to 4 weeks | **YIELD:** approximately ¾ cup

INGREDIENTS

* ½ cup dried herbs or 1 cup fresh
* 1 cup neutral oil or enough to cover herbs (I prefer organic olive or jojoba oil for most uses.)

Instructions

1. If using fresh herbs, allow to wilt for 24 hours to reduce moisture content and thereby prevent mold growth in your oil.

2. Fill a mason jar three-quarters full with chopped herbs.

3. Cover the herbs with oil, poking with a chopstick or knife to release air bubbles. Be sure to add enough oil to cover the herbs by a minimum of ½ inch above the plant matter.

4. Tightly lid your jar and gently shake, and then place on a saucer in sunny windowsill, shaking your jar daily or anytime you think of it. Allow to steep for 3 to 4 weeks. Always check that your herbs are completely covered with oil after each shake. If the herbs soak up the oil and you have trouble submerging them at any time, just add a bit more oil to your infusion.

5. Strain the infusion through a clean, dry piece of cheesecloth, squeezing to extract as much goodness as possible from the herbs. Store your infusion in a clean, dry, labeled jar for up to 1 year.

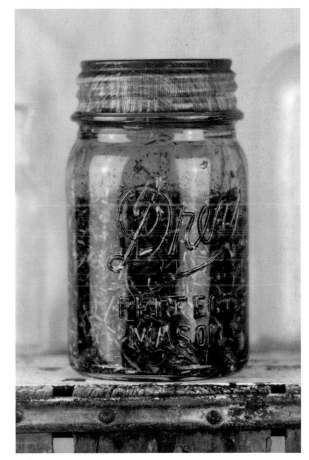

BASIC STOVETOP-INFUSED OIL

Stovetop-infused oils are high-quality infusions that come together much faster than the solar method. Though I appreciate the unhurried process of solar infusions, stovetop infusions are ideal when time is a concern. Speed for the win!

ACTIVE TIME: less than 20 minutes, not including foraging and wilting or drying time
TOTAL TIME: 24 hours or more | **YIELD:** approximately ¾ cup

INGREDIENTS

- ½ cup dried herbs or 1 cup fresh
- 1 cup neutral oil or enough to cover herbs (I prefer organic olive or jojoba oil for most uses.)

Instructions

1. Place your herbs in a small, nonreactive saucepan and cover with oil.

2. Gently warm your oil and herb mixture until quite warm but still well below a simmer. (A double boiler works well to prevent overheating.) Cover and remove from heat and allow to sit until cool.

3. Repeat this process several times, allowing the herbs to infuse for a minimum of 24 hours before straining. The longer—and slower—you steep, the better your infusion quality will be.

4. Strain the infusion through a clean, dry piece of cheesecloth, squeezing to extract as much oil as possible from the herbs. Store your infusion in a clean, dry, labeled jar for up to 1 year.

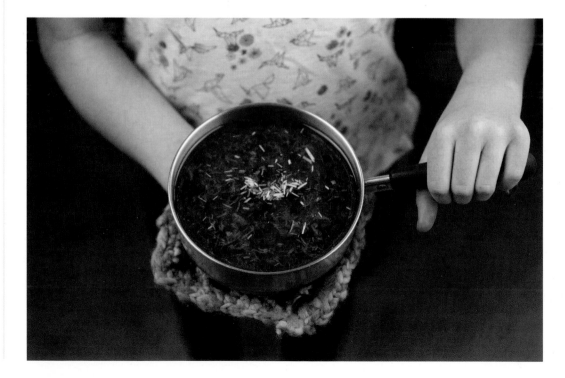

RESOURCES

Organic Herbs and Beeswax

If you are unable to forage or purchase herbs locally, buying online is a wonderful option! Mountain Rose Herbs is my favorite source of certified organic herbs, beeswax, and other ingredients: www.mountainroseherbs.com

Packaging

Reuse packaging you already have on hand by washing and drying tins, jars, and lip balm tubes. If you'd like to purchase new packaging, Sunburst Bottle is a good source with no minimum order size: www.sunburstbottle.com

Additional Books

Eager to learn more? Here are a few of my favorite books about herbs.

Just for Kids

Herbal books for kids are a rare treat! My own kids have thoroughly enjoyed the following:

Walking the World in Wonder, by Ellen Evert Hopman. Healing Arts Press: 2000.

Herb Fairies series, by Kimberly Gallagher. CreateSpace Independent Publishing Platform: 2015.

Herbal Recipe Books

The books listed here are excellent places to find even more recipes (for kids and parents alike).

Medicinal Herbs: A Beginner's Guide, by Rosemary Gladstar. Storey Publishing: 2012.

Herbal Recipes for Vibrant Health: 175 Teas, Tonics, Oils, Salves, Tinctures, and Other Natural Remedies for the Entire Family, by Rosemary Gladstar. Storey Publishing: 2008.

Foraging

My favorite foraging books are written for adults.

Identifying and Harvesting Edible and Medicinal Plants in Wild (and Not So Wild) Places, by Steve Brill. William Morrow Paperbacks: 1994.

Incredible Wild Edibles, by Samuel Thayer. Foragers Harvest Press, 2017.

Kitchen Herbalism

These books are a rich source of information about the healing power of food. Written for adults.

Alchemy of Herbs, by Rosalee de la Forêt. Hay House: 2017.

Eating on the Wild Side, by Jo Robinson. Little, Brown and Company: 2014.

Technical Knowledge

Excellent resources for someone wanting to dig deep in their understanding of herbs, their uses, and contraindication. Very technical but useful references for adults.

300 Herbs: Their Indications & Contraindications, by Matthew Alfs. Old Theology Book House: June 2003.

Making Plant Medicine, by Rico Cech. Herbal Reads: 2016.

The Earthwise Repertory, by Matthew Wood. North Atlantic Books, 2016.

DEDICATION

To my dad and his (seemingly ceaseless, occasionally tiring, childhood-long) game of "*what tree is that?*" which changed the trajectory of my life; to my mom, who has demonstrated time and again that it's never too late to follow your dreams (keep writing, you!); to my sister Leah, who has shown me how strong and capable one woman can be; and to my husband and best friend, Pete, who has stood beside me and cheered me on, dream after dream after dream after dream. You are one in a million, babe.

Most of all, this book is dedicated to my kids, Sage and Lupine. You, who can hear the plants whispering, inspire me daily with your curiosity, wisdom, and intuition. This is the book I wanted when you were young. (In its absence, I named you after plants. *I hope that isn't weird.*) Love, Mama

GRATITUDE

So many hearts, heads, and hands have coaxed this book into life. How grateful I am to each person who helped this project take root (a fraction of whom are mentioned below)!

To my husband, Pete, and our children, Sage and Lupine: for your patience as you sidestepped herbs, medicine-making supplies, and photo spreads throughout our house for months on end; for tirelessly stepping in as needed for photographs and recipe testing; and for picking up the slack around the farm while I was busy writing. And—most importantly—for making time for this project in our lives. You gave so much for this book to come to fruition and I am deeply grateful. I think it's time for ice cream.

To my editor, Thom O'Hearn, for reaching out to me with the concept for this book, and quickly setting the pieces in motion that allowed it to take shape; and to Amanda Soule, for inviting me to write for *Taproot Magazine* and welcoming me back to those pages again and again. Thank you both for being resources for me throughout this process and holding my hand as I learned the publishing ropes for the first time.

To my sister, Leah Jepson, and my herbal student and friend Allie Brandon, for your mad proofreading skills; and to my neighbor/herbalist/mentor/friend Jess Krueger for checking my work with your keen herbalist's eye.

A special thank you to the tireless troupe of local families who welcomed me into their homes or met me out in the fields and forests of the Driftless for the photographs that grace this book: Amanda, Soren, Fox, and Finley Caldwell; Jaali Parrish; Sonya, Cecil, Addisu, and Lina Newenhouse Wright; Jody, Ava, Lilah, Jude, and Lucy Bendel; Heather, Willa, Sabine, and Livian Roth-Amodt; Jonel, Iris, and Mae Kiesau-Gorrill; and Laudy Schulz. How honored I am to have your friendly, familiar faces looking back at me from these pages!

And a heartfelt thank you to the parents and kids of Green Magic Summer Camp 2017. Our weekend together was the seed that germinated and grew into this book. And what fun we had! For all of your enthusiasm, feedback, and joyful participation, I am deeply grateful.

To Lucky Nielsen of *Happy Go Lucky Creations* for your magical illustrations (Herbal Paper Dolls on page 137.); Ginny Sheller, Ray and Kelly Syler, and Sarah Lee for your last-minute photo rescue missions; neighbor Alan Slavick (our favorite tinkerer and a fountain of plant knowledge) for pausing your prairie restoration work to allow me time for photos and foraging; and to elderberry man Mike Breckel for our photoshoot amidst your glorious plants.

And finally, I offer humble thanks both to the countless plants who so selflessly share their gifts with us, and to the herbalists who generously share their work and knowledge that we may learn and grow from their wisdom. My inspiration comes from many, including Rosemary Gladstar, Matthew Wood, Matthew Alf, Jim McDonald, Rosalee de la Forêt, John and Kimberly Gallagher, Susan Weed, Jess Krueger, and Mary Glick.

INDEX

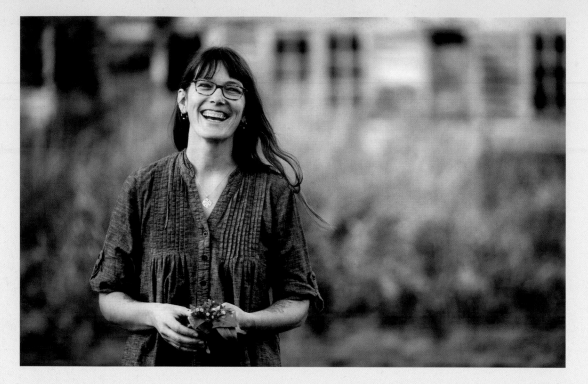

ABOUT the AUTHOR

Rachel Jepson Wolf loves nothing more than bringing people and plants together. With a degree in environmental education and biology, Rachel spent years helping kids and adults fall in love with the natural world. In 2002 she founded LüSa Organics, a botanical body care company, and more recently began leading in-person herbal retreats for adults and children.

Today Rachel lives with her husband, Pete, and their two children, Lupine and Sage, on a wonderfully weedy homestead in rural Wisconsin. Her days are spent writing, foraging, playing with plants, and homeschooling her kids. Find Rachel online at www.rachelwolfclean.com, where she blogs about herbs, farm, and family; or explore her herbal body care line at www.lusaorganics.com.

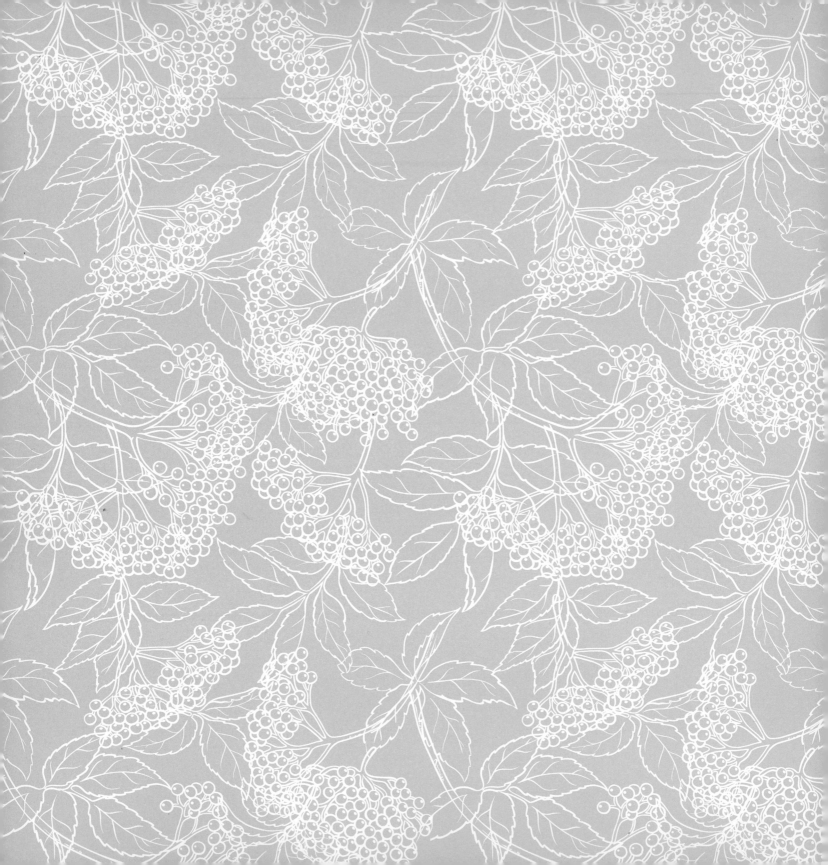